Get Back Into
Your Jeans Diet

Also by Monica Grenfell

5 Days to a Flatter Stomach

Fabulous in a Fortnight

For details of how to order these and other Pan Books, please see page 182.

MONICA GRENFELL

Get Back Into
Your Jeans Diet

PAN BOOKS

First published 1999 by Pan Books
an imprint of Macmillan Publishers Ltd
25 Eccleston Place, London SW1W 9NF
and Basingstoke

Associated companies throughout the world

ISBN 0 330 37303 X

9 8 7 6 5 4 3 2 1

A CIP catalogue record for this book is available from
the British Library.

Exercise photographs by Lesley Howling
Typeset by SetSystems Ltd, Saffron Walden, Essex
Printed and bound in Great Britain by
Mackays of Chatham plc, Chatham, Kent

Contents

Acknowledgements

This book is dedicated to my two wonderful sons, Michael and James Lavers, who are always so supportive and encouraging.

I would also like to thank all the people who took part in the diet testing and Tesco Stores plc for their help in supplying food information.

My particular gratitude goes to Gordon Wise at Pan Macmillan for his patience, enthusiasm, diplomacy, energy and skill as my editor, and for making it all such a pleasure.

Introduction

The Keys to Getting Back Into Your Jeans

Wouldn't you just love to be able to get back into your favourite jeans by this time next month? Or be a dress size smaller? Wouldn't we all! Well, with this plan you can – and you'll also discover that this is the last diet you'll ever need. I have written books on the best diet for a flatter stomach – *5 Days to a Flatter Stomach* – and the best diet for beauty – *Fabulous in a Fortnight* – and now I am going to give you the most successful diet I have ever devised – the ultimate weight-loss plan, whether you use it for a quick fix or to get you started on a whole new life of slimness.

This diet is foolproof. You're going to go down one dress size in a month, and you're going to feel sensational. If you can add up a column of figures you can lose weight successfully, just like the hundreds of elegant, glamorous women I advise every year. The old days of feeling washed-out, hungry and eating second-rate food are over. The past few decades have been littered with faddy diets, diets which ban a huge range of foods, diets which restrict fat or protein, or combinations of foods, diets which have had you lying awake half the night, hungry – and worst of all, diets which just didn't do anything for you. Well, on this diet you'll eat great food and still lose weight.

This is not a cosy plan which has you sitting back while I tell you what to do. I don't preach, but nor do I fool you that it is easy to be slim. It takes effort, and your input needs to be pretty high for the next month. But it's worth it. This is a campaign: you're going to grit your teeth and go for it, and once you've gone down a size you can carry on and lose another. There's an exercise plan and records to keep (see pages 101 and 65–67), but that's the beauty of it – you can't go wrong because *you* are in the driving seat.

I have called this book the *Get Back Into Your Jeans Diet* because experience tells me that most of us see weight loss in terms of wanting to regain a certain image. It's not just your body which bothers you, but how you look in your clothes. You've probably got fond memories of times when you felt good and looked good, and those memories are usually linked to clothes. They may have been your wedding dress, a special suit or your bikini, but they stay in your wardrobe as a benchmark. Gaining weight or losing your figure can mean more than just throwing out a few clothes which have become too tight. It can mean losing your identity. 'I just want to get back into those jeans!' has become such a familiar cry from my clients and the people who write to me that I decided to make it the title of this book. It also helps to point out that a good diet should be for *everybody* – I have as many letters from men as from women on the subject of weight loss and fitness, and most men are just as concerned about their health and appearance as women.

Mind you, weight loss is only part of the story. We all want to look *good* in our clothes and that means not just less fat, but toned muscles too. You might have lost half a stone, but what's happened to your stomach? And can you really bare your thighs on the beach, slim as they are?

You talk about losing your figure and wanting to get it back. Your figure is as much a part of your personality as the colour of your hair or your name. You own it. Size and shape are two of your main defining features. They matter, and in this book I am going to tell you how you can learn to shape up for good.

• • • • • • • • • •

Something For Everyone

Have you ever noticed that most diet books contain pages and pages of reasons to diet, quizzes and questionnaires, testimonials and recipes, and just a few pages of what you are actually going to *eat*? Well, this book is the exception. I have given centre stage to what you really want to use a diet book for – different diets, ideas and suggestions to suit you, whatever your situation, like my snacker's diet, and plans for those with intolerance, arthritis and ME. You'll find meals suitable for the whole family, vegetarian alternatives, 'gourmet'-style menus and, of course, a few 'cheap and cheerful' ideas. And, you know what? They are all devised from the same range of food. It's amazing how inventive you can be even if you are given just seven basic foods and a piece of fish or meat to plan around. I want to prove to you that there's a diet out there to suit everyone – and this is it!

I'm on a diet. It's not a weight-loss diet, but it's maintained my weight at the same level for fifteen years. It's based on porridge, bread, fruit, cheese, salads and meat. I've also cut out sugar. It works because these are the foods I love and the ones I've got rid of are the ones I'm not bothered about. You'll find your own diet, too, thanks to this book. *I promise.*

'Men Don't Fall for our Fat Ratios'

In *5 Days to a Flatter Stomach* I pointed out that men don't fall for women's 'fat ratios', whatever slimming magazines might have us believe. A good figure and bags of confidence are what get you noticed. No one looks at you across a crowded room and thinks, 'She looks like she weighs nine stone, so she's the one for me.' They either like what they see – or they don't. If you feel awful being a size or two larger than you should be, you'll probably lack that crucial confidence. What I'm going to help you to do in this book is to regain your confidence. It makes sense!

• • • • • • • • • •

But That's All About Losing Weight, Surely?

If you've weight to lose, yes, but you might be happy with your weight and unhappy with your shape. Most people have one bit of them which is out of step with conventional clothes sizes, and if you sit down all day you're likely to have poor muscle tone. Others need to lose a lot of weight before they can even consider exercising. I know one very large woman who can't walk more than one hundred yards without feeling shattered, so her first priority is to get her weight down.

Take the long view. You must have been a size 10 once. You're simply on the first rung of the ladder to getting back down to it. But start now, and make it a job that you want to do well.

Will There Be A Lot Of Exercise?

Up to a point. If you're the type of person who is well used to your nightly fix of aerobics, this will be a doddle. However, if you're never seen out of your armchair after 7 p.m., it'll be a shock. But likely as not you need to make exercise more of a permanent fixture in your life anyway. It shouldn't be something you 'fit in'. But nor do I want it to be something that you endure, or which bores you rigid.

One of the secrets of weight control lies in re-programming your body to expect both a certain amount of food and exercise, so a commitment to the exercise programme, together with the food plan, is a must. Weight fluctuations will be a thing of the past once you understand that exercise isn't just a way of 'working off' what you've eaten. When you get to the section on 'homeostasis', this will make more sense (see pages 29–31).

Nobody was ever sorry because they went for a walk. Nobody ever felt worse for a stretch. Try to adopt the attitude that it's a necessary part of your goal. You can achieve a lot with diet, but it won't improve your shape.

• • • • • • • • • •

I've made it simply for you by mapping out a realistic exercise programme which most people can manage. Your goals are clearly set out so that you know when you've done enough. You are aiming to burn extra calories through exercise and to reduce your calorie intake by about 300–500 calories a day, depending on your personal calorie allowance (see pages 44–45). This adds up to a lot in a week, and the more exercise you do, the more weight you will lose.

No time for exercise? I don't believe you. Everybody has twenty-four hours in a day, and we all have more time than our grandmothers. If you have a washing-machine, you have time. If you have a car, you have time. If you ever sit for more than an hour each day watching television, you have time. If you value your figure, want to start afresh and make something of yourself, then you must *make* time. And I hate to say this, but *you* put the weight on in the first place. Eating less takes no time at all, and all the time you save from eating less can be spent in going for a walk! You'll never regret it.

I'm not talking about a vigorous regime which has you getting out of bed at five in the morning for fifty press-ups. And I'm not going to suggest that you leave the car at home and walk three miles in the rain just to lose half a pound. Yet if big thighs are your problem, they aren't going to disappear simply by wishing them away. Leg lifts and bottom squeezes, and stomach crunches, waist whittlers and hamstring curls, oblique twists and hip stretches are all part of my daily repertoire of exercises that keep my clients toned and trim, and admired by all their friends. I'm not saying we enjoy it, but who enjoys sitting at the hairdresser's with chemicals spread all over her hair? Yet we'll put ourselves through that expense and inconvenience a thousand times if it makes us look good. That's how you must approach your exercise routine: it's worth it, and the pay-off comes later. That pay-off being when you ask the assistant to fetch you a smaller size, or you make it back into your jeans.

• • • • • • • • • •

So What's The Secret About This Diet?

It's understanding the brilliant way in which carbohydrate
foods control your appetite and your moods. Carbohydrates,
such as potatoes, rice, bread and fruit, are all miracle foods
when it comes to weight control, and you'll never feel the same
way about food again once the diet starts to 'kick in' to your
system. People who are lifelong bingers and food fanatics tell
me that on this diet they went for a whole day without wanting
(or even thinking about) sweets or chocolate; how they came
near to lunch-time and didn't even notice; how they thought
there was so much food on this diet, yet their weight continued
to fall. And most of all, I have letters galore from diehard
weighing fanatics saying they have not even thought of the
scales for a month.

The other secret about this diet is counting calories. It may
sound boring, but there's nothing dull about losing weight and
having everyone admire you. The alternative is staying as you
are and never wearing those jeans again – and you don't want
that. The best thing about calories is that no foods are banned,
just monitored, and the main aim of this diet is to have you
losing weight *safely*, *healthily*, and *effectively*, which means
keeping it off for good.

You also need to restrict added sugar in your diet. Once you
do that, which will automatically cut down on the range of
foods you consume anyway, your weight will fall – not dramatically, but gradually. Yes, I know you want to lose a lot of
weight quickly, but this way you will never gain weight again.

You will have to restrict your food intake and there's no
easy way of doing that apart from willpower. But if you lack
willpower I am going to give you all the motivation I can! You
will succeed. Not only that, but your weight will remain steady
for the rest of your life. You won't be weighing yourself at
every opportunity because you'll find you don't care. You'll
look good, and you *can* get back into those jeans! Once you

• • • • • • • • • • •

learn to balance your energy equation, the simple system whereby calories *out* exceeds calories *in*, you can lose weight, stay slim and still enjoy your meals.

I've Been Watching My Fat Intake – What About That?

Watching fat intake seems to work for some people, but it's not the Holy Grail in itself. The nation eats less fat than it did sixty years ago, yet obesity is at an all-time high. Why is this? Years ago people ate less food and therefore fewer calories, and they took more exercise. They also planned their week's menus and bought what they needed, and not what took their eye. You had to ask for items, unlike today when you trundle round the shelves and pick up whatever takes your fancy. It is better to monitor fat by eating less food, and to eat foods which don't contain fat, than to eat fat-reduced foods such as yoghurts, biscuits and cakes. My own informal research has shown that instead of forgoing biscuits and cakes, people are actually choosing the lower-fat variety, thereby eating more than they mean to. I get so many letters from people who say they are not losing weight on a 'low-fat foods' diet that I can only conclude that they are still eating too many calories.

Fat intake looks after itself on this diet because there is very little fat in basic foods. Since you only eat one or two protein foods – such as fish, eggs, nuts or meat – fat is automatically cut there too. Your only task is to keep records of your food for a month. After that, it will become second nature.

People often say that they don't want to be bothered with weighing out food portions and counting calories. Then, in the next breath, they talk of their despair about their weight. They say that they can't be bothered fiddling with food diaries, but they think nothing of spending an hour cooking, eating or bingeing on food which makes them ill. Fine then, stay as you are! I don't want to sound mean, but there's effort involved in achieving anything. If you're tried everything else and it hasn't

• • • • • • • • • •

worked, why not just give this a go? I have provided suggestions for all the menus for you (see pages 138–78). Stick with the main menus and devise all the permutations you like.

The Beauty Of Carbohydrates

When I was young, carbohydrates were seen as stodgy and fattening, and best avoided when you are on a diet. We all kept slim by strict regulation of food intake and were hungry all the time. My main foods were fruit and salads. The day started by worrying about what I was going to eat, and if I managed to eat very little I was pleased with myself. The more hungry I got, the better I liked it, and if I succumbed to a biscuit offered at a friend's house, I felt like a failure. Headaches and tiredness were a part of life and the price I had to pay to be slim.

Does this sound like you? What makes me sad now is that I missed out on so much. I am exactly the same weight now as I was then, yet now I eat what I like! Yes, I'm careful and I never, ever 'pig out' because I don't believe you can get something for nothing in the weight war, but it worked once I understood what's called the 'glycaemic response'. Don't switch off at this point, because the glycaemic index is actually quite interesting, and it's all happening right inside you. When you eat a meal, you're provided with energy in the form of calories. Digesting, absorbing and metabolizing breaks the food down into cells that your body can use. Blood-sugar levels are at their highest half an hour after you've eaten and they return to fasting level after 1½ to 3 hours. The quicker the glucose is absorbed into the bloodstream, the quicker the level falls again. The slower it is absorbed, the slower the rate of return. So food which takes time to enter the bloodstream also takes time to leave it, and you therefore have more energy, for longer.

Blood-sugar levels should be kept constant to maintain a level of alertness and energy. If they fall too low, you recognize the familiar symptoms of lack of concentration, sleepiness and a general weakness or lassitude. The only foods which give instantly available energy are carbohydrates.

Carbohydrates include sugars, starches and fibre. You may think that all sugars are rapidly absorbed into the bloodstream and therefore have a high glycaemic index, but they don't. Natural sugars, such as those found in fruit and milk, have a *low* glycaemic response, which means that they enter the bloodstream slowly but keep the sugar levels steady for the longest time. Added sugars, such as those found in chocolate, sweets, squashes, cakes and biscuits have a *high* glycaemic response. They enter the bloodstream very quickly to raise sugar levels and give 'instant energy', such as a chocolate bar consumed before playing football, but levels soon fall dramatically, due to what is known as the 'insulin response'. Insulin is secreted in the body to keep sugar levels from becoming dangerously high, but its presence forces sugar to become so low that you feel tired again quite quickly. Unless you have a proper meal, the result can be a continuous yo-yo effect of high and low blood-sugar levels.

Starches, found in potatoes and rice, also have a high glycaemic response, but fibre-rich foods, such as apples, pulses, dried fruit, pasta and cereals, have a low glycaemic response. It is important to eat a combination of the two and to keep added sugars to the very minimum in any diet. Only by having a steady blood-sugar level can you hope to beat food cravings and binges, and the beauty of carbohydrates is that they are filling and satisfying. If you are in any doubt about the important part that carbohydrates play in meeting your energy levels, compare the amounts of protein, carbohydrate and fat needed each day by the average person weighing 10 stone (63.6 kg):

- Carbohydrate   254 grammes
- Protein   48 grammes
- Fat   70 grammes

An important part of this diet is the restriction of added sugars. In the medical and dieting world not much has been made of the true part played by sugar – partly, I think, because it is not linked to any major disease. However, unlike fat, added sugar is one food for which your body has absolutely no need. The only reason it is added to food is to make it taste better, although it thereby encourages a 'sweet tooth' (and not very good ones, either!). Personally, I think this is terrible. Man isn't meant to eat sweet food, except for naturally sweet things, like fruit. By cutting out sugar, you will automatically reduce your calorie intake and gradually lose weight in a painless way. If you eat a diet that is rich in complex carbohydrates, control your portions and embark on an exercise plan. You will soon find that you can go for days without needing your old sugar 'fix'. Here is my promise to you if you continue this plan for a month:

- You will stop bingeing and craving food
- You will never have fluctuating weight again
- You will not wake up and step straight onto the scales
- You will not worry about every mouthful, every social event and every pound
- You will not care about your weight, only your size.

You are going to lose weight, go down a whole size and get back into those jeans. You will never look back! I really understand how to control weight. This is my ultimate weight-loss plan and I am confident of its success for you.

• • • • • • • • • •

Back To Basics:

Your Body Has A Mind Of Its Own

You can only begin to understand weight control when you can understand why you store fat in the first place. Forget fancy diets which say that you can't mix some foods, or tolerate others. Man is a hunter, designed with the ability to eat massive quantities of food in one go, as available, and to mix anything with everything, storing most of it as available energy and saving the excess as fat for harder times.

Today, despite the easy availability of fast food and little danger of starvation in developed countries, we are still the same animals, and eating more than we need means that we store fat. This is a perfectly normal human function. Some people wonder 'What's gone wrong?' when they start to gain weight. Nothing's wrong. Your body is simply doing what comes naturally with the fuel that it doesn't immediately need.

Mother Nature has only one thing on her mind – the survival of the species. However, what Nature doesn't know is that if you are a woman, you may have decided not to have children or you may have already completed your family. As far as your body knows, if you are fertile, you need stores of fat, regardless of any pregnancy. Fat stores are usually positioned around the hips, stomach and thighs. This is why women have greater trouble in losing fat from the lower body, although fat stores can be anywhere on the body, including the back, arms and chin!

Your body doesn't know that it isn't always going to have to sustain a pregnancy, or to hang on for a few days until the

● ● ● ● ● ● ● ● ● ●

next meal is available. So it still stores fat in case of need. But this doesn't mean that your body doesn't know best. If you place your body under starvation conditions by crash dieting, or being on a continual diet of too few calories, you will be on a permanent seesaw of weight gain and loss. Later on in the book I will explain this in more detail. In the meantime, it is important that you understand the processes which govern our metabolisms.

Never put your body into 'starvation' mode by going for hours or days without sufficient food. Listen to its pleas for food and nourishment and act on the signals. Your body has a mind of its own. If you treat it badly, it will pay you back in terms of yo-yoing weight gain and loss, moodiness, irritability, depression and failure. Listen to your body: it deserves better than this.

• • • • • • • • • •

My Foolproof Way to Lasting Slimness

Does this sound familiar? For years, you've dieted without success. There's nothing you haven't tried. The result is always the same. During the first week you lose 5–8 lbs (2¼–3¾ kg) and then you get stuck. Your friends seem to eat anything they like and still stay slim, never gaining so much as an inch or a pound. You tell yourself you know the reason why: you have a slow metabolism and other people just burn calories off faster than you do.

I'm afraid you're wrong. The correct reason for this is that you aren't active enough, and you probably eat more food than you think. You may not eat much, and you've probably been watching fat content rather than calories, but even a fat-less diet can be loaded with calories. In terms of energy burning, the key to weight loss is the calories. For example, a 98 per cent fat-free bagel has 235 calories. Twenty-five grammes of jam (one ounce), which is totally fat-free, contains 70 calories. Boots low-fat flavoured yoghurt probably has 155 calories. On a calorie-restricted diet you can find that these figures soon mount up to a calorie count that is well over your basic needs, and being just a few calories over the limit on a regular basis soon leads to the sort of weight gain that you find baffling. I get a lot of letters through my weekly Sunday magazine column which say exactly the same thing: 'I seem to have put on a stone in the past year and I don't know how. I'm eating the same as I always did, but the weight's creeping on.' It's very upsetting, but people don't realize how these little differences can add up to a big difference over time, especially if you aren't exercising.

What Are calories?

Calories are the units of energy that fuel all forms of life. They are essential to keep you alive and not eating is like trying to drive a car with an empty petrol tank. The only problem comes when you eat more calories than your 'tank' holds. It's then that you become fat.

Counting calories is a foolproof way of managing your weight because you know straight away if you have exceeded your intake. What you need to keep an eye on is the *Energy Balance Equation*. This means balancing your energy *input* (what you eat) with your energy *output* (how much you burn off).

There are three ways to balance the energy equation:

1 Eat fewer calories than you burn off.
2 Eat the same amount of calories and increase your level of exercise
3 Increase your exercise levels and decrease what you eat.

You will lose weight and even change shape successfully on this diet because:

1 Weight control is based on calories in versus calories out
2 You will be calculating your own calorie requirements
3 *No* food is 'unlimited' – this theory only adds calories and is a misleading 'reward'
4 You won't be counting misleading fat grammes and eating low-fat foods which can actually *make* you fat because you're eating more of them, and they're full of 'weight-sticking' additives.
5 You will avoid the high-fibre foods which can cause bloating.

• • • • • • • • • • •

But If I'm Calorie-counting, Will I Become A Calorie 'Junkie'?

You certainly shouldn't. However, you might worry that once you start focusing on the calorie content of food, you will be carrying around a calorie reference book for the rest of your life. Don't worry. You will soon get to know roughly how many calories are contained in what sort of foods, and after a while it will become second nature. I bought a calorie-counting mini computer a while ago, which told me how many calories I was burning in daily activities. At first I wore it all the time. I was so fascinated I couldn't take it off. How many calories was I burning off during my keep-fit class?; how many calories were shed in that walk round the village?; how many an hour at my word processor? After a while it got crazy. But I soon realized that most days evened out to about the same. I also found that I wasn't using as many calories as I thought I was, and I adjusted my food intake accordingly. You'll find you won't be counting calories for ever, because you won't need to.

When you look at a calorie booklet and think that you'll never remember all those values, remember: you won't be eating all those foods! We all have our favourite foods, so you only need to know the ones that you eat most of the time. You will soon learn that a jacket potato has about 200 calories, a quarter of a medium-sized pizza contains 290 calories and an apple has 50. And you will look at a helping of cottage cheese and be able to guess its quantities pretty accurately, given what you already know. Very soon you will have a 'sixth sense' about it all. You won't become a calorie junkie because, with a little thought, you won't need to be.

• • • • • • • • • •

Your Questions Answered

Why Does My Weight Keep Fluctuating, And Why Do I Gain Weight So Easily?

I receive hundreds of letters every month, and I see dozens of clients. If there is one theme that recurs time and time again, this letter really says it all . . .

'Please help me. I am twenty years old and have always been overweight. By July 1995 I weighed 11½ stone [69 kg] which was the final straw. I started exercising and cutting down on snacks. My weight gradually fell and when I started university it kept on falling because I began an aerobics class as well. By March 1997 I weighed 9 stone 4lb [56 kg] and was a size 14.

'I was looking and feeling great. There were several times when I had a binge, but due to the aerobics I managed to maintain that weight. Then during summer break this year, my weight went back up to 9st 12lb [59 kg]. I was paranoid about the other weight returning and went on a stupid diet with a friend who advised me to eat only one 'healthy' meal a day and to exercise. I took this to an extreme in order to reach my goal of losing a stone [6 kg] in a month. My daily food intake consisted of one bowl of cereal for breakfast, an apple for lunch and just boiled rice with vegetables in the evening. I also overdid it with the exercise, doing two hours every day. I felt very tired, but stuck to it. I was overjoyed at the end of the month when I weighed in at 8st 12lb [53 kg] and took a size 10–12.

'But from that day on I began bingeing out. Sometimes I felt out of control, eating up to six slices of pizza with chips, cakes and chocolates in one sitting. To make up for this, I starved myself the next day.

'Six months later, I weigh 10 stone [60 kg]. I have been strict with

• • • • • • • • •

myself, trying to allocate realistic lifetime targets that I can maintain even after weight loss. I go to aerobics three times a week, always walk around instead of driving and take the stairs wherever possible. I am a chocoholic but have resisted the temptation so far. I eat cereal for breakfast, fruit and a sandwich for lunch and have spicy foods in the evenings. I have been following this routine for the past three weeks but my weight has nonetheless increased to 10st 3lb [61.2 kg].

'I just don't understand where I am going wrong. At times I feel as if I am going crazy. The first thing I think about before doing anything is how much I can eat and what to eat, and this obsession is driving me crazy. I can't seem to concentrate on anything. I just want to be 9 stone [54 kg]. I have tried everything, but all the weight is on my stomach and 'love handles', and I have gone from a size 12 to a 14–16. Every time I set myself a target I find I just give up because it doesn't work any more. Please help me!'

Anita, Glasgow

The problem here is essentially one of chaotic eating and a lack of control. In Back to Basics (see pages 11–12), I talked about the logic behind nature's need to store fat. However, in the normal course of events, nature is not so stupid as to store so much fat that it slows you down. Regular, frequent eating also reassures your brain that your body is always going to be fed. The point is to control the intake.

I can best describe the impact of chaotic eating on your body by asking you to picture a parallel scenario which you probably wouldn't contemplate: try sleeping for three hours tomorrow morning and two hours the following afternoon, then skip the following night's sleep altogether and make up for it by having twelve hours the next day. Then deprive yourself of all sleep for a solid three days. How do you think you would feel? Exactly.

People who regularly have erratic sleeping habits get out of sorts and find their bodily functions become out of step. Yet many of us, including Anita, expect our bodies to cope with constantly changing eating patterns. Piles of pizza, chips and chocolate followed by a day of nothing. Wild aerobics for three weeks with calories severely restricted, followed by mountains of food and no exercise at all. In the middle of this nightmare she expects her body to lose weight. Well, the body doesn't actlly respond to a day without food by shedding – or using up – fat. On a strict diet like the one that Anita followed for a month, hours were passing without her consuming any food at all. In this situation the body's only response is to shut down its systems to save as many calories as possible, which is one reason why she felt so tired. The body can store between 1,600 and 2,000 calories at a time, which is generally used up in the course of a day, but as these stores become depleted you begin to feel weak and lethargic.

On this kind of diet what you won't do, however, is to use fat. Yes, Anita lost weight, but at least half of that was glycogen and water, two of her body's most vital components. Her actual fat loss, I suspect, was very little and it was inevitable that she not only gained back the weight, but also binged madly because she missed eating, and her body was worried that it might never see food again. In such circumstances the metabolism slows down considerably to save fuel and this is why weight is always regained at such an alarming rate.

You *must* get into a routine! Lack of routine is one of the main reasons why people become fat. When I say 'chaotic' eating, I don't mean grabbing a sandwich for lunch, or occasionally skipping breakfast. I mean dieting and bingeing like Anita. A binge is eating for the sake of it, saying 'to hell with it' as you clear up after guests and finish off the trifle and cheese just because it's there. A binge is what you feel you need when you've been on a diet but broken it by having a slice of cake, and you then hate yourself. You feel guilty, so you buy a chocolate bar on your way home and eat it because now you might as well. You probably have it in the back of your mind that you'll start afresh tomorrow, so you might as well eat while you are still in the mood.

Bingeing is a frame of mind. It comes on when you have deprived your body of nutrients, and chemically it is screaming out, sending instinctive messages to the brain. Bingeing happens when you feel the damage is so bad, you might as well add to it. It is one of the causes of weight gain and is brought on by chaotic eating.

Anita will beat her problem when she learns to take a longer view. She must start now and get her confidence up. Anita must stop weighing herself constantly, start to eat four times a day and give it three months at least. If she follows the advice in this book, her weight problems will never return.

On this plan you will say goodbye to bingeing and starving by following a frequent-eating, carbohydrate-loaded diet. You'll get back into your old jeans by next month and never look back!

Why Do I Get Food Cravings?

Food cravings are your body's cry for help. To understand them, imagine a really raging thirst. What does it make you want to do? You have to have a drink. Now, think about being really cold. What does this make you want to do? You put on extra layers. And what if you are terribly hot? You take off some of your clothes or go somewhere to cool down. Sensations, such as thirst, are hard to describe and you don't always know where they come from, but they are irresistible. They make you do exactly what you must in order to prevent a life-threatening situation – in this case, dehydration. Hunger, cold and heat are also life-threatening situations and your body forces you to do something about them by providing a sensation to which you respond. Feeling an irresistible urge to eat is the same kind of force. Your body needs nutrients which you are not giving it and it therefore provides the urge. It is as simple as that.

One of the most common cravings is for magnesium, another is fat. It may not surprise you to learn that both of these are contained in chocolate! People who are on strict diets are very likely missing their magnesium intake, so they are the most likely to binge out on chocolate and fatty foods, thus keeping the crave–binge–starve cycle going. I should also add here that chocolate contains caffeine, and caffeine is highly addictive. People who talk about getting their daily chocolate 'fix' are, in fact, craving caffeine, as well as magnesium and fat. What's unfortunate is that chocolate also contains a lot of calories per bar. If you're in any doubt that fat is a major source of craving for the human body, ask yourself when you last saw someone bingeing on broccoli, or chicken liver or fresh crab meat? How about lentils and tomatoes? We all know the jokes about pregnant women's cravings, but under normal circumstances we just don't binge on those foods. Instead, we binge on mountains of buttered toast, whole pizzas, chips and chocolate gateaux. It happens most of all when a diet has been too low in fat and calories due to a desire to lose weight in the fastest possible time. *Fatless diets cause cravings and binges*.

The other reason why we binge is low blood sugar. If you insist on skipping breakfast and you eat very little during the day, you will crave sugar. Sugar enters the bloodstream very quickly and provides instant relief for tiredness and hunger, but the downside is that it triggers off what is known as the 'insulin response'. Insulin is secreted in your body to prevent your blood sugar from going dangerously high, but it also provides too much in anticipation of a further meal. If a meal doesn't come along, your blood sugar will be low and this results in a feeling of weakness and lethargy.

The way to beat irresistible cravings is to eat regularly. However, you have a weight problem which is bothering you

• • • • • • • • • •

and food is obviously a culprit, so is it right to say that you 'need never feel hungry' on a diet?

I don't believe so. It was a dislike of hunger and a liking for food which got you to where you are now, and hunger is not bad in itself. For example, if you are going out for a special meal in the evening, might you not enjoy it all the more for having worked up a real hunger for it? There's a difference between being hungry because you're trying not to eat – which is *bad* – and being nicely hungry for your next meal, and this is what you must learn on your new plan. Don't listen to people who tell you you need never do without your favourite foods or be hungry if you are to lose weight successfully: you do. But you are doing it sensibly, retraining yourself and developing your most precious asset – WILLPOWER! So start now, establish a routine which fits in with your life and stick to it. And follow these golden rules:

* If you have a big meal one evening, *don't* get up the next day and skip breakfast and lunch to make up for it. Eat your meals as you would have done normally so that your body learns to trust you. Knowing that you will have to eat the next day may also stop you from overeating in the first place.
* Don't starve yourself all day just because you have a special event to go to in the evening and are thinking that you are bound to overeat. Have your usual meals. If you suspect a high-calorie feast is in the offing, compensate for this by cutting down on portions at your usual meals, such as one piece of toast instead of two, a salad instead of soup for lunch, etc. *But don't eat nothing at all!*

You will find that regular eating banishes cravings. If you are a lover of 'fattening' foods, remember that *no* foods are fattening in themselves. It is the calorie content and your intake that matters. For example, four apples have more calories than 25g

• • • • • • • • •

(loz) of chocolate (if that's all you eat!). A main meal salad contains more calories than a small portion of chips. Eat a variety of foods, incorporating what you like but maintaining a balance; eat regularly and you will stop craving food.

Why Is My Friend So Slim When We Both Eat The Same Things?

This has a lot to do with your genetic tendency to store fat in certain parts of the body. My family, for example, all store fat in the upper body which leads to double chins and spare tyres! The only saving grace we have is that we hardly ever get fat legs or bottoms. A common mistake, though, is to believe that a tendency means an *inevitability*; it doesn't. Never mind that your aunties and your cousin and your three sisters all have fat thighs, it doesn't mean that you will too. My family don't all have double chins, but that's the first place where my weight goes.

We all envy other people's tiny waists or thin thighs, but the fact is that no one was born with a God-given ability to eat just anything they like and not gain weight. If your friend eats a lot and is slim, it simply means that she's using her fuel and you aren't. There's always a reason. Look at the section on calorie burning and exercise (see pages 101–104), and you will see how changes in ordinary everyday tasks (such as washing a car instead of going through the car wash) can make a lot of difference to your calorie burning.

Which Foods Are Fattening And Which Ones Aren't?

No food is fattening and no food is slimming. It's all down to how much you eat of it. I have already talked about calories and cravings, and the fact is that if you are a 'chocoholic' you *should* include some chocolate in your daily diet. Remember though, that chocolate is not as healthy as fruit, and the fruit should be there too!

• • • • • • • • • •

Fat yields nine calories per gramme, as opposed to protein and carbohydrate having four calories per gramme, hence you can eat more of these without gaining weight. Simply remember that all foods have the potential to cause weight gain if you eat more than your body needs.

Too much sugar makes you feel lack-lustre and irritable. Sugar causes the 'insulin response' as explained earlier (see pages 9 and 20), but many people respond to that by having *more* sugar! Being fed a constant supply of sweets, chocolate bars and fizzy drinks, without pausing for a square meal, your appetite is constantly dampened and you don't give your body the chance to get properly hungry for a really good meal. Blood sugar levels swing wildly and the effect on your moods can be dramatic. Just ask any diabetic!

My next ban is on junk food. Too many additives are simply not good for you or your digestive system. Pure, fresh food is a *must*. If you take a little time to prepare food, this also means that you may think twice about what you eat instead of just cramming in something you've microwaved in a minute.

Don't think of any food as being fattening. It is how much you eat of it which is fattening. If you want to lose weight, cut down on portions. Ration yourself to weights and amounts. Don't just snack, even on endless amounts of fruit and vegetables, just because you think it's not fattening. Get into overall good habits with food – it is not your enemy!

How Can I Stop Picking In The Evening?

You don't need to. You may not believe it, but evening eating is not outlawed on my diet, nor should it be. There is a lot of rubbish talked about late eating going to fat, and it's a fallacy. I have already talked a lot about routine and if your routine is one of evening eating, then carry on. Remember that many people, such as professional actors and dancers, not to mention shift workers, have to eat late. They aren't all fat!

• • • • • • • • • •

However, there's a world of difference between 'picking' in the evening and eating an evening meal, and you shouldn't be doing both. Picking at food when you are not hungry comes down to basic boredom and habit, and the best way to stop this is to save your meal for as late as possible (within reason), and to make sure that it is not too fatty, too sweet or too large. For example, it is not a good idea to have a main meal *and* a pudding, unless that pudding is fruit or a light mousse-type dessert.

In an ideal world you should make breakfast your biggest meal, your midday meal a reasonable size and your evening meal very small – but life isn't always like that! Most of us race around in the day and snatch a sandwich if we're lucky, and what could be nicer than relaxing in the evening with a good meal and possibly a glass of wine? It's not quite the same thing, gazing over the candlelight at a ham sandwich! Here are the golden rules about late eating:

- Don't have a full roast and two veg. Meat takes about eight hours to pass through the system and you won't sleep well if your body is working hard to digest it.
- Don't eat fried food, or food which is too sweet, late at night.
- Make room for a late snack by eating a lot less earlier on.
- Try not to eat later than 10 p.m.
- Do not have heavy sauces, such as cheese sauce, white sauce or sauce with cream in it. Pasta sauces made with vegetables and tomato sauce are lighter and more digestible.
- An ideal meal would be potatoes with fish and vegetables or salad. If you just want a snack, try toast or cereal with fresh fruit.

The best way to manage evening eating is to exercise first. Go to a fitness class or the gym, or have a brisk walk or run on summer evenings. Perhaps you might spend the evening gardening? All these activities are ideal for evening eaters because the body uses food more effectively when it is taken *after* exercise when your muscles are restocking themselves. I think of it being like bare shelves in a supermarket after the Christmas rush. You need to stock up again quickly, ready for the next rush of customers!

How Can I Raise A Slow Metabolism?

How do you know that your metabolism is slow? Is it because you gain weight so easily? And just what is metabolism anyway?

It is the rate at which your body burns its fuel and it is rather like an engine. A Rolls-Royce uses a lot of fuel because it is so big and heavy, but a Mini uses little fuel because it is small and has an uncomplicated engine. Your metabolism depends on the following:

- Your age
- Your weight
- Your gender
- The amount that you eat
- The amount of muscle on your body
- The amount of exercise that you take.

Let us look at each of these in turn:

Your age

Your body weight is a mixture of everything contained inside you, so it won't surprise you to learn that putting on weight doesn't necessarily mean that you've gained fat. Weight is also muscle and your metabolism is muscle-driven.

If you're gradually losing muscle because you're getting older – and who isn't? – your metabolic rate will also decrease. It isn't a lot over a year, but it starts from the age of about twenty-five. By the time you've reached forty you're possibly just beginning to notice what started years ago, and it's called 'middle-age spread' – fat stored around the middle which our slowed-down metabolism isn't dealing with any more. If you add to that a natural tendency to slow down as you get older, to become more placid and less easily upset, or maybe the chilren have left home so there's less running around, or perhaps you've been promoted to a more desk-bound job, or retired so you aren't working at all and/or you have fewer money worries, then it can seem as though you've suddenly gained weight at the age of forty-five. In fact, the process began about twenty years ago!

Remember, ageing is not just something that happens to people who are older than you are. *Even if you are eighteen, you are still ageing. Take steps before it becomes a problem.* The secret to keeping abreast of metabolism changes is to *increase the amount of exercise that you do for muscle strength*, thereby keeping up your muscle size, and to *increase the amount of aerobic activity that you carry out.*

Your Weight

I have already talked about the difference between a Mini and a Rolls-Royce when it comes to fuel consumption. When you weigh a lot, your body will need a lot more fuel to keep it going. If you weigh very little, your resting metabolic rate will be a lot lower.

Your Gender

Men have a higher resting metabolic rate than women because they have a greater proportion of muscle on their bodies. It doesn't necessarily mean that a man has a higher capacity for exercise, and a man who sits at a desk all day will have an inferior endurance to a woman who keeps fit on a regular basis. But on the whole, women do have 80 per cent less active muscle than men and they store more body fat. It won't be much comfort to women for them to know that in the event of starvation, they will survive longer than men, but the fact remains that the higher proportion of body muscle in men means that their metabolism is slightly higher.

The Amount That You Eat

The body does a lot of amazing things in a week:

- Your heart beats more than 700,000 times
- You breathe more than 121,000 times
- Your stomach produces almost five litres of digestive juices
- Your entire outer skin cells are replaced
- Your hair grows about two millimetres
- I,750 gallons of blood passes through your kidneys.

And to think that some people do this on a diet of next to nothing!

All these functions – and many more – happen even if you are asleep and on top of them you have your daily life with its stresses and strains. We all have what is called a 'Basal Metabolic Rate' (BMR). This is the number of calories that are needed to keep all your basic processes going, even if you were to lie in bed all day doing nothing at all. It's the reason why a person still needs to be fed, even if he is in a coma. Your BMR depends on how big a body you have and how much muscle, and it's fair to calculate your resting BMR at about a calorie – or just under a calorie – for every minute of the twenty-four-hour day. On pages 44–5 I have given you an easy way to calculate your personal BMR.

The process of eating *raises* the body's metabolic rate because digesting food requires energy. If you eat frequently, there is always something going through your system, so that it won't shut down to starvation levels. When I was at school, there was an old wives' tale that we teenage girls used to trot out about a boiled egg being worth 'minus' calories because it took more calories to digest than it actually contained. I think it was probably a bit of an exaggeration, but even so there was a grain of common sense in the theory. Certain foods require a lot of energy to be broken down by the body, and hard-boiled eggs, high-fibre foods and meat are just three of them. The basic point is that digestion uses energy and starving yourself requires none.

The Amount Of Muscle On Your Body

You can weigh 54 kilogrammes (9 stone) of muscle or 54 kilogrammes (9 stone) of fat. Most of us are a mixture of both. Naturally slim people often eat little and take no exercise, and as they get older their lack of muscle tone not only leads to weakness and injury, but also weight gain. By keeping good muscle tone your metabolism is raised and you can enjoy food without gaining weight.

The Amount Of Exercise That You Take

The best type of exercise for increasing your metabolic rate is muscular strength work. Next comes aerobic exercise. Exercise should be vigorous and last for more than forty-five minutes. The general medical advice is to do a minimum of twenty minutes' hard exercise three times a week for health purposes, but if you are young you can easily manage forty-five minutes. And the best reason for exercising vigorously is that it uses up your body's glycogen stores which are then replenished after activity. It should take only two minutes for your heart rate to recover after strenuous exercise, but your blood pressure and metabolic rate stay high for up to two hours afterwards, which makes it the best time to eat. Your metabolic rate is also higher, even when resting, if you have been working at improving the tone of your muscles.

• • • • • • • • • •

A final word about exercise. Talk about the muscle fat ratios, 'strength training', 'resistance training' and 'endurance' can be off-putting if you're new to exercise. It sounds as if you'll be weight lifting and running marathons, and it conjures up pictures of you sweating away in a gym or squeezing your hips into a tight Lycra leotard! Well, it doesn't have to be any of these. The activity can be anything from combing your hair to vacuuming the carpet to pruning the roses. Strength training is anything that requires muscular strength, such as heaving furniture, digging the garden or cycling. Endurance is anything you can do for a long time, like going for a couple of hours' walk. If there is one message that I want to get across it is that exercise is anything that you want it to be, and it needn't cost anything.

Why Have I Suddenly Gained All This Weight?

Many people who have been slim all their lives ask me this when they find that their 'normal' weight seems to have increased. If you've never needed to worry about your weight, it can be very upsetting. You're following the same routine and living the same life, yet the weight is piling on – or is it? When I investigate clients who complain about sudden weight gain, it's usually happened over a long period of maybe a year. It's all down to a process called 'homeostasis', which is the body's ability to regulate itself over a period of weeks and months, rather than hours or days. It is the body's overall ideal functioning state of balance and applies to all your functions – your salt–fluid balance, for example, or your sugar levels, or your hormone levels. Your general weight is also subject to this balance, so although most of us fluctuate by a few kilogrammes either way, there is usually a mid-point at which your body is happiest.

When your weight is usually steady, a weekend's heavy eating won't make any difference at all. If you starve yourself for a day, then it won't make any difference either, and any

• • • • • • • • • •

weight loss is soon regained. We all know that it is possible for the body to lose a lot of weight very quickly, say in the case of a jockey or boxer who has to register at a certain weight to qualify for competition. I know of one jockey who 'lost' 4.5 kilogrammes (10 pounds) in weight in just four hours by taking diuretics tablets which made him lose fluids rapidly, but this wasn't his 'true' weight, of course. (It's also not at all good for your body's system, and I'd advise against taking diuretics as part of any weight-loss plan.) As soon as his race was over and he had had a few cups of tea his body retained them and his weight shot back up again by 4.5 kilogrammes. This is homeostasis (see below) working! The body has remarkable ability to maintain balance, and you've got to work with it. These extreme measures make no difference to your shape and size, so if you want to start afresh, get slim – and get back into those jeans – you need a different approach. You need *routine, regular meals* and *exercise*.

The Miracle Of Homeostasis

Here's how homeostasis works in practice. Say you were used to a ten-minute walk to work and back every day for years and you gave up work to have a baby. A major part of your routine will have been altered. It may have seemed like nothing in comparison with all the other changes, but twenty minutes of walking, five days a week for forty-eight weeks a year, is eighty hours of walking. It takes 24,000 calories of fuel to achieve this, doubtless mopping up a good amount of your excess intake! On top of that, what if you used to have just coffee for elevenses every day and now you have two biscuits with it? Again, it doesn't seem much for one day, but if this becomes a routine then you have added 500 calories a week or 26,000 calories a year. With the loss of the outlet of 24,000 calories and the additional 26,000 calories, this equates to a whole stone (six kilogrammes) in weight!

• • • • • • • • • •

The point is, having the odd couple of biscuits won't change your weight, and forgoing your daily walk for a few days won't make any difference either. However, the problem arises when you give up one routine which is firmly embedded and take on another. Weight 'creeps up' on us because we don't take these little changes in food and exercise into account – but your body does. Your body becomes programmed to your routine and will stick with what it knows, unless you start to reprogramme it with a new routine. Many young mothers find that their weight changes for the worst when they stay at home and they find it baffling because life is so hectic. It is also demoralizing to feel unattractive and fat, but keeping busy is not the same as being active. Physical activity is what burns calories.

You let weight creep up on you by not paying attention to the little things like exercise and the odd cake or biscuit. Soon you have relaxed your standards and 'let yourself go'. The good news is that the process also works in reverse. This diet plan will get you back into good habits and hopefully make you aware of how to balance what you are eating in terms of extra food and how that relates to activity for the rest of your life.

Influencing homeostasis is a way of setting a computer programme. As we know, people who have been used to crash dieting find that whenever they start to eat normally again, they gain weight. This is natural, but if you wait and let your new programme lodge itself into your system, your weight will soon fall again. Exercise is subject to this control too and when you start a new exercise programme it may take a few weeks before you notice a real difference. *But it will happen!* Just sit tight, stick with the plan, watch the calories and let nature take its course.

Getting Back Into Your Jeans

How Does This Diet Work?

Let's just recap on where we've got to so far. Weight problems and failing to manage your weight at the end of a diet are caused by:

- Eating too many calories
- Eating chaotically
- Failing to plan meals
- Not using up all the calories that you eat
- Not eating enough carbohydrates
- Lack of willpower.

Here is how you are going to deal with these challenges:

1. Eating too many calories

You will soon be calculating your own daily calorie requirement (see pages 44–45 and 71). You write down the total calorie allowance and simply deduct calories as you consume them.

2. Eating chaotically

Chaotic eating means reaching into your office drawer for a sandwich, eating in the street, eating whilst you're preparing food and eating at odd times. This leads to weight gain. *The only way to successfully beat the problem is to retrain yourself.* It sounds harsh and you probably feel as though you're being treated like a child, but trust me. On this plan you'll be making mealtimes and sticking to them. You'll schedule everything, even your snacks or cups of tea. Believe it or not, although you'll start by thinking about your next meal and gasping for the next snack, your frustration won't last. You've probably got an unbalanced approach to food right now which is why those jeans or that dress won't fit, but in the long run, your new habits will bring you a lot of happiness – and clothes that fit!

3. Failing to plan meals

In the hustle and bustle of daily life, you probably lurch into a supermarket and wait for inspiration to strike. I've done it myself. The biggest problem about this approach is that it leads to what I call the 'pineapple syndrome'. This is an old joke in our household. Many years ago, I bought a pineapple because it was reduced in price. I was in a hurry, I hadn't a clue what we were going to eat, and I was casting around the shop for inspiration. I shoved the pineapple in the fridge and then forgot all about it. Two weeks later I found it and a stab of guilt flashed through me as I fought my desire to chuck it out straight away. It's good food, I thought. I'm sure I can do something with it.

Half an hour and five recipe books later, I settled on a Pineapple Upside-down Pudding. The only problem was, I didn't have half the ingredients, so I drove to the shops, paid to park and fought my way around a packed supermarket. Back home, hot, tired and irritable, I cooked up the cake. The kitchen looked like a bomb-site and there was a mountain of washing-up. On producing it proudly for the family, my elder son declared that he couldn't eat another thing, my younger son asked didn't I know, he hated pineapple? and my husband said he thought it looked a bit heavy, but he'd have a go. I burst into tears and ended up eating three helpings just to get rid of it.

• • • • • • • • •

Feeling fat, and much later on, I actually chucked what was left of the whole sorry mess onto the compost heap.

You've probably done something similar to this yourself. I went shopping without a clear meal plan and bought food in the hope that something would come out of it. Not only is this strategy a complete waste of money, it'll also make you fat. Like buying food to have 'in case someone pops in' (they never do) unless you're the sort of person who can throw food out without a twinge of conscience, you really must make meal plans in the future. On this diet, you'll know what you're going to buy before each week starts.

4. Not using up all the calories that you eat

As you have already learned, calories need to be used in activity. If you're not losing weight, you'll need to increase your exercise.

5. Not eating enough carbohydrates

On this plan you will be choosing at least *seven* portions of carbohydrate every day, four of which will be fruit. These will be chosen from a set list.

6. Lack of willpower

You do have willpower! You want to get back into those jeans or that dress, and you are reading this book. All you have to do now is to keep that goal firmly in your mind.

On this plan I have taken the basic decision-making out of your hands by restricting the range of food available. From there, you can either make up your own meals or you can go with some of my menus. Your willpower will be needed when it comes to raiding the biscuit tin, refusing second helpings and picking at food which you are preparing, but *you have the willpower*. Don't be afraid of hunger while you look forward to your next meal. Don't be tempted to snack. You won't be ill because you already have energy stores there – right on your hips or stomach or thighs! Every time your tummy rumbles and you think you just can't bear it, think of that bit of fat disappearing. If you give in and eat those crisps, the fat will stay exactly where it is. It's as simple as that. Use your willpower and keep your mind focused on those jeans – how loose they're going to be!

What Will I Be Eating?

The idea is to choose from a list of foods which are also portion-controlled. For example, this may be two slices of bread or 100g of pasta, two slices of crispbread or two apples. Each unit counts as one choice and you can choose a total of seven units a day. Turn to page 75 to see your first week's menu.

The units are calorie-counted for you and you tick them off in your food diary as you eat them. In addition, you can choose one or two extra protein units from another list which go on to make up balanced meals. It sounds complicated, but it isn't. Once you get used to the idea you won't ever have to keep a food diary again. By counting calories, keeping your sugar intake low and your complex carbohydrate intake high, you will retrain your body and mind into a healthier, more balanced way of eating which brings lasting success in the weight-loss battle.

Making It Easy For You

If I have learned one thing over the years, it is that whatever diet I devise, I can't please everyone. However, most people ask me to set out their meals for them to take away the stress of decision-making. Maybe you are extremely busy or pressured at work, perhaps you have so many people to cater for that you find planning meals too complicated? I will show you how easy it is to be inventive with these food lists. You can either go with my suggestions or plan your own menus.

It doesn't matter whether you're a gourmet, vegetarian or harassed parent, male or female, young or not so young, we all want to get back into those jeans – and stay in them for good! In addition to the food lists, there are five other rules:

1   *No* ready-packaged, supermarket convenience meals as you won't be able to tailor their contents to your requirements
2   *No* alcohol, except on your day off
3   *As little* added sugar as possible – use sugar-free products wherever you can
4   *No* diet colas, 'low calorie' yoghurts or desserts, or other artificially calorie-reduced products
5   Eat *seven* portions of carbohydrates every day

You can choose any vegetables from the long list on page 54. They are not free of calories and you must still deduct them from your daily allowance, but you can make your own selection.

Have one day off from the diet every week. This is important because the diet is a strict regime from which you need a break every so often. However, on your free day, resist the temptation to eat as much as you can from all your banned foods! Food is *never* a treat. Don't use it as a reward. It's no reward to put your weight back on again and then feel depressed. Remember: the taste of any food only lasts a couple of minutes. *Looking slim lasts a lifetime. The reward is in how you feel about yourself, and how good you look.*

Carbohydrates

Carbohydrates are your most successful diet foods. They are divided into two groups:

Complex*	Simple**
Bread, flour, wholegrains	Sucrose – fruit and vegetables
Pasta	Lactose – milk, yoghurt, etc.
Rice	Fructose – fruit, honey
Vegetables	Maltose – barley, grains
Pulses – peas, beans, etc.	Glucose – vegetables, fruit, honey.

* Complex carbohydrates raise the blood-sugar level slowly. Their energy lasts for several hours and they can be used as a base for many meals. About 1,600–2,000 calories can be stored at any one time.

** Simple carbohydrates raise the blood–sugar level quickly, but energy levels fall quite quickly.

Proteins

After water, protein is the most plentiful substance in the body and it's absolutely vital that you eat enough of it. Think of the wear and tear of living, and how it takes its toll on you. You have worries, you have stresses, you have relationship problems. Your children may be driving you mad, or perhaps you work in a pressured environment. Because of these problems, your immune system takes a battering and the hormones which affect your metabolism, weight and sexual activity are also undergoing constant repair, maintenance and renewal. Only protein can help to repair the damage that has been caused. Typical signs of protein deficiency are falling-out hair, brittle nails and rough skin. You may also suffer from tiredness, anaemia and depression.

Types of Protein

There are two types of protein – complete and incomplete. To be complete, a protein has to have eight amino acids, which are classed as essential. They cannot be made by the body and have to be eaten in our food. The best sources of complete proteins come from the following:

• • • • • • • • • •

- Fish
- Meat
- Eggs
- Milk
- Dairy products

Some plant proteins are high in quality protein, although they can never be as good as animal proteins. These include:

- Soya beans
- Brewer's yeast
- Nuts
- Seeds
- Wheat germ.

If you exist on a diet that is made up entirely of plant proteins, you will risk protein deficiency. If possible, always try to include at least one complete protein in a meal – cheese, or an egg or milk for example – in order to benefit from maximum good health.

Too Much Protein

Despite what I've said about how essential it is to eat enough protein, your body doesn't need it in huge quantities. As a rough guide, you need about three-quarters to one gramme per kilogramme of your body weight every day. One example of this amount of protein is that the average person weighing 64 kilogrammes (10 stone) would require just 48–64 grammes of protein per day which can be found in one chicken breast and 568ml (one pint) of milk.

Too much protein is counter-productive because it can't be stored in your body. Excess protein also makes your urine acidic, which leads to a loss of calcium, and most westerners eat far more protein than they actually need. As a guide, if

● ● ● ● ● ● ● ● ● ●

you're consuming meat, 568ml (one pint) of milk, a cheese sandwhich and an egg breakfast every day, then you are eating too much protein – and far too much saturated fat!

On the other hand, if you are trying to lose weight, it's all too easy to eat too little protein. Living off salads, fruit and vegetables, with just the odd piece of bread or slice of ham, will definitely not give you enough protein and, in time, you'll feel pretty awful. Whether you are studying, working, managing a family or whatever, few of us lead lives that allow us the leisure to feel washed-out half the time – and you'll also look so bad!

How Much Protein Do You Need?

To work out your weight in kilogrammes divide your weight in pounds by 2.2, e.g. 11st 2lb equals 70.9 kg. Then multiply 70.9 kg by 0.75, which equals 53.18. Therefore if you weighed 70.9 kg, you would need 53 grammes of protein a day.

If you are particularly active or sporty, or if you are recovering from an illness, or you are pregnant, increase this to one gramme a day per kilogramme of your body weight. You'll find out exactly how many grammes of protein are contained in foods by studying food labels. For example, 568ml (one pint) of milk equals 3.2g protein, 125g spaghetti equals 10.8g protein.

Fats

You can always tell a person who is obsessed about cutting out fat in their diet because their skin looks dry and flaky. And, as I've already explained, one of the reasons why you may occasionally go berserk and eat everything in sight is because you're eating too little fat (see pages 12–13 and 19–22). It's important to be careful about saturated fats, though, and good as it is, your intake of animal produce *must* be monitored for the sake of your heart. Choose lean meat, don't eat fat or crackling and drink skimmed milk wherever possible. In the weight war, even the so-called 'good' sources of fats, such as those found in nuts, seeds, olive oil and fish, can make you fat if you have too much of them. However, oils found in these foods are brilliant for your health and looks.

For this diet, I have included a special cake recipe (see page 144), which includes lots of lovely seeds and dried fruits. This will be a real treat and it will help give you the fats you need.

Once you start eating the right amounts of fats you should find that your food cravings vanish and this will be a major breakthrough in the weight war.

A word of warning about 'fat-reduced' and 'fat-less' claims: the general move in the food industry to reduce fat content is undoubtedly good. The problem comes, though, when people eat fat-reduced food when they might otherwise have eaten nothing at all – or too much of it, as they think they have more leeway. I have actually heard a fellow shopper saying she didn't want any crisps, then changing her mind when a certain label caught her eye. 'Oh, I could have these low-fat ones, instead,' she said. Instead of what? Instead of not having anything at all?

Don't be fooled: even healthy food can contain a lot of calories. If you're going to win the weight war, you must take note of calories from *all* sources.

Sugar

For years, my job as a diet counsellor has been to keep beautiful women slim in the face of gruelling schedules and constant entertaining. I devise personal diets for them and my low-sugar or sugar-free diet has always been one of the most popular and successful.

On the *Get Back Into Your Jeans Diet* your added sugar intake must be cut. Natural sugars are already found in many

• • • • • • • • • •

foods, such as milk and vegetables, and we could not function well without them, but added sugar is totally unnecessary for your body. You should cut it out altogether.

On average, each person in Britain buys and eats 40 kilogrammes of sugar every year. Even if you think you don't eat a lot yourself, you may not have a choice. Half of the sugar that you eat is 'hidden' – added in by some food manufacturers to enhance flavour. This all adds up to the obesity and weight troubles of the nation, and, in my opinion, it is a scandal that is not taken seriously enough. Sugar rots your teeth and adds 'empty' calories to your intake – ones you can't use. There are just three main foods with empty calories: Sugar, Lard and Alcohol. Watch out for them!

Twenty years ago I used to diet like a maniac. I was always hungry, but I was also slim. I was constantly tired and washed-out – but I was slim. It all seemed as if it was worth it, but I didn't count sugar as one of the main reasons why I felt so exhausted – instead of eating sensibly I was using it for a boost. My diet biscuits couldn't be so bad, I thought, that low-calorie chocolate bar was fine, and I could fill up the rest of the day on fruit. However, I slept badly and, quite frankly, was a different woman. I decided to cut out added sugar to keep my son company when he was suddenly diagnosed as being a diabetic, and I have never looked back. Today, without the aid of supplements or tablets of any kind, I have the energy and vitality to work a sixteen-hour day, and my figure is better than it was when I was twenty-five. Finding sugar-free alternatives is easy, and you can lose your sweet tooth altogether, especially if you keep up your carbohydrates.

There are two types of sugars: *extrinsic*, which means sugars that are not naturally present in food as they have been added, and *intrinsic* sugars, which are part of the food. Examples of these are as follows:

• • • • • • • • •

Intrinsic (no restriction)	Extrinsic (limit to 60g a day)
Milk	Table sugar
Starches	Jams
Fruit	Biscuits
Vegetables	Cakes
	Sweets and chocolate

How Much Sugar Do I Need?

The World Health Organization recommends a daily intake of added sugar to be no higher than 60 grammes a day (or 10 per cent of your total calories). So, on a 1,500 calorie-a-day diet, you should eat no more than 150 calories of sugar.

Foods With 'Hidden' Sugar

Here are some examples of typical foods with added sugar – before they even get to you!

Coco Pops (per 30g serving)	12.0g sugar
1 slice chocolate Swiss roll	20.5g
Seafood sauce (per 100ml)	14.6g
340g Chicken Vindaloo	13.9g
Ready-made coleslaw 100g	5.8g
Cheese and pickle sandwich	12.5g
Standard 290g can cream of tomato soup	15.6g
Nutri-grain 98 per cent fat-free	12.0g

As a comparison, here are some ways of cutting sugar:

Shredded Wheat 30g serving	0.1g sugar
Profiterole (with cream and small chocolate topping!)	3.9g
dsp home-made mayonnaise	1.3g
Tandoori breast of chicken	3.0g
100g home-made coleslaw	1.2g

• • • • • • • • • •

Roast beef or chicken sandwich	1.2g
Regular bowl fresh lentil soup	1.7g
Go-Ahead Chocolina (each)	3.4g

Making the Right Choices

Always study food labels as these give precise information about carbohydrate and sugar contents, as well as other nutritional values (see also page 46). The big retail chains have recently introduced new labelling which shows at a glance into which category a product falls:

Sugar-free	Contains no added or natural sugars
No added sugar	No sugars added from any source
Low-sugar	Less than 5 grammes of sugar including those naturally present
Reduced sugar	At least 25 per cent less sugar than the standard product – but beware, as the original product may have had a lot of sugar in it in the first place!

It is easy to make the right food choices. *Take control of your diet. Don't let anyone else load you with unwanted calories.* The first two categories are really the ones to look out for – but remember, don't buy or eat something just because it's low in sugar or sugar-free: keep track of the calories as well.

Counting Calories

As you have already learned, the amount of calories that our bodies need is highly individual. Your BMR (basic metabolic rate, see page 27) depends on factors such as age, gender and starting weight, so diets which recommend a set number of calories per day are not ideal. I have devised many such 'universal' diets myself over the years and whilst they serve their purpose, I think it is better to give you several different

• • • • • • • • • •

menu plans from which to choose to suit your own calorie requirements.

The service that I offer to my clients is a personal one. We spend the time working out exactly what they need and keep revising their calories week by week. Much as I'd like to, I can't do that for you, so I've done the next best thing: I have tried to offer so many different options and calorie counts that you should find yourself catered for. Some of the menu plans are quite low-calorie – less than 1,000 per day – while others go as high as 1,600 calories. As a rule of thumb, you should stick to the less restrictive limits the more weight you have to lose, and the longer you have been overweight, but if you are simply trying to lose the few kilogrammes that you put on over the holidays, or to shape up before Christmas so that you can fit into those party clothes, then you'll be quite safe to go for the more immediately lower-calorie diets.

To start, multiply your weight in pounds by nine *or* multiply your weight in kilogrammes by twenty. The two figures at which you arrive are hardly different. This gives you your resting metabolic rate although you can go a little below it if you aren't able to take much exercise – for example, if you are desk-bound, or suffer from a medical condition which means you cannot be active.

Now, you may be in the region of 90 kilogrammes (15 stone) or more, so by this reckoning your daily calorie total would be 1,890. Sorry, but it's not! The formula doesn't work 'ad infinitum', and I'll explain why. The heavier you are, the more weight you have to move around – *in theory*. But if you are very heavy you aren't going to go for the same jogs and half-hour walks, and running up the stairs and games of tennis as a lighter person. It's no shame, because by reading this book you're doing something about it. However, even though they *will* be, your calories aren't being used just yet.

The top limit is 1,600 calories for everyone over 72 kilogrammes (12 stone). Don't feel bad if you're way over this weight. I admire you for doing what you're about to do, and success will be all the sweeter when you achieve your goal, for having overcome something that was such a problem for you. You're going to stop feeling bad, you're into a new phase of your life and you're going to be *successful*.

Revising Calories Downwards

As you lose weight, you need to revise your calorie allowance downwards, or increase the intensity of your exercise plan (see page 121). If you've been on diets before, you'll know that depressing 'plateau' stage which nearly everyone experiences. This is where you stay the same weight for two or three weeks, despite being very strict with yourself and not cheating. I'd say that half of all dieters give up at this stage, and it's understandable. After all, it's one thing to be exercising iron willpower and seeing results, but quite another to be denying yourself and *still* not losing anything.

Rather than eating less, which I am not at all happy about because you need your nutrients, I would prefer to see you exercising off an *extra* 200 calories or so to keep up the weight loss. Don't groan! 200 calories is easily used up in a forty-minute walk, forty minutes of housework, twenty minutes' swimming or fifty minutes of shopping! And don't forget that you will also gain the benefits of better muscle tone and circulation, which is far better than if you were to simply cut your food down and sit in front of the television.

But My BMR (Basic Metabolic Rate) Gives Me More Calories Than You Specify In Your Menus!

Lucky you! You can simply make a higher calorie choice from the proteins list and have two choices instead of one. And don't forget, you don't *have* to use up your full calorie allowance or be worried about getting the figures precisely right. Fifty calories over won't matter too much, but neither should you go hundreds below your limit in the hope that it'll help you to lose weight faster. It will, but the weight will come back on just as quickly, I promise you. Never forget your goal – you want to get back into those jeans, and you want it badly enough. The taste of that cake will last a couple of minutes. *It's just not worth it.*

Reading Food Labels

Counting calories and finding out how much sugar is in your food is not as hard, time-consuming or as fiddly as you may think. Yes, at first it takes a bit of concentration and effort, but soon you will be able to glance at a label and know instantly whether it is the right food for you. Knowledge is power: I used to find I had been eating some things for years without realizing just how bad they were for me!

As I've already explained, two most important pieces of information for following the *Get Back Into Your Jeans Diet* are carbohydrate and sugar content. Here is an example of a typical food label from a breakfast cereal:

Nutrition Information

Typical values	Per 100g	Per 30g serving
Energy	387kcal	116kcal
Protein	6.5g	2.0g
Carbohydrates	85.5g	26.0g
(of which sugars)	49.0g	14.7g
Fat	1.0g	0.3g
(of which saturates)	0.2g	0.06g
Fibre	3.0g	0.9g
Sodium	trace	trace

• • • • • • • • • •

There are three very important pieces of information contained here. First, the fat content is low and the *saturated* fat content is extremely low at only 0.06 grammes per 30 grammes – the size of a typical bowlful of this particular cereal. However, this information can be slightly misleading when it is used by slimmers on their weight-loss plans. Note that the added sugar content is 14.7 grammes per serving, nearly *three times* the sugar content of many sugar-free cereals. As you will also be counting carbohydrates on this diet, the information that this cereal contains 26 grammes of carbohydrates is also useful.

It's worth mentioning too, that the lower-fat content of this particular cereal does not mean it is low-calorie. It has sixteen calories *more* per bowlful than sugar-free cereals. It may seem a bother to read labels and count calories, but you won't mind when you see your thighs getting slimmer and your bottom becoming smaller – and when you get back into those jeans that you've always dreamed of wearing again!

Vitamins

What do they do?
Vitamin requirements vary according to lifestyle and age, but we all need the right balance of vitamins to feel well and to function properly. For example, lack of iron makes you feel tired and breathless, while lack of vitamin C can lead to aching joints and sore gums. Children need more vitamins than adults simply because they are still growing and developing, but it is also possible to overdo it. Excess vitamins and minerals can cause their own problems, and for further details you should consult a good natural health reference book. But this shouldn't be a reason not to take sensible doses of supplements when you are eating a good diet.

What vitamins can't do is give you energy. Many people feel

that a spell of tiredness and stress, and especially feelings of weakness and lethargy, can be overcome by popping mega-doses of pills. It doesn't work like this! Vitamins do *not* give you energy – they don't have any calories! Only calories can give you energy and, as you have already learned, calories come from food. You see, you do need the right ones!

Ideally, you should gain all the vitamins and minerals that you need from your food. But good reasons to take extra vitamins may be in times of great stress, illness, pregnancy or lack of appetite, when nutrients could be missing from your diet, or your condition may be draining you of nutrients. *Never use pills as a substitute for food, but as a supplement.*

Here is your guide to the essential vitamins, where to find them, how much you need – and how much is too much! If in any doubt as to your own needs or restrictions, consult your doctor.

The Essential Vitamins

Vitamin	Where Found	Symptoms of Deficiency	Symptoms of Excess	Daily Requirements
Vitamin A	Cheese Kidneys Eggs Butter Fish oils Apricots Peppers Carrots	Fragile bones Loss of appetite Sight problems	Hair loss Headache Vomiting Defects in new babies	50g carrots or a slice liver
Vitamin B1	Potatoes Kidneys Beans Peas Cereals	Swelling limbs Confusion Muscle weakness Loss of sensation	None known	4 tbsp rice or 6 slices wholemeal bread

• • • • • • • • • •

Vitamin	Where Found	Symptoms of Deficiency	Symptoms of Excess	Daily Requirements
Vitamin B2	Chicken Fish Meat Milk Eggs Cereals	Cracked lips Bloodshot eyes Skin problems	None known	1 bowl cereal
Vitamin B6	Cereals Nuts Bananas Yeast Eggs Soya beans	Deficiency is rare	Nerve damage to hands and feet	1 bowl cereal or 1 portion fish
Vitamin B12	Meat Chicken Dairy products Fish	Tiredness Pins and needles	None known	1 glass milk or 1 portion fish
Niacin	Peas Beans Sweetcorn Nuts Cereals Potatoes Meat	Tiredness Skin rashes Diarrhoea Depression	High doses could result in flushed skin	1 piece fish, meat or chicken
Folic Acid	Spinach Broccoli Cereals Watercress Bread	Wasting of the gut because nutrients cannot be properly absorbed	None known	2 portions vegetables or 4 glasses orange juice
Vitamin C	Potatoes Apples Citrus fruits Vegetables	Aching joints Fatigue Sore gums Pain in the bones Loss of appetite Scaly skin	Excess is mostly excreted in urine and mega-doses can cause disturbed sleep	1 orange or potato

Vitamin	Where Found	Symptoms of Deficiency	Symptoms of Excess	Daily Requirements
Vitamin E	Wheatgerm Nuts Seeds Vegetable oils Margarines Fish oils	Deficiency is rare	None known	30g nuts

Minerals

We all need a wide range of minerals to maintain health and for the following bodily functions:

- Strong bones and teeth
- A healthy immune system
- To enable vitamins to work.

The Essential Minerals

Minerals	Where Found	Symptoms of Deficiency	Symptoms of Excess	Daily Requirements
Calcium	Milk and other dairy products Sardines Sesame seeds Green leafy vegetables	Muscle weakness Back pain Soft and brittle bones	Loss of appetite Vomiting Constipation	800–1000mg
Magnesium	Wheatgerm Beans Peas Nuts Sesame seeds Figs	Tiredness Weakness Cramps Chocolate cravings	None known	

• • • • • • • • •

Minerals	Where Found	Symptoms of Deficiency	Symptoms of Excess	Daily Requirements
Potassium	Avocados Bananas Fresh and dried fruits Beans Peas Mushrooms Tomatoes	Extreme thirst Weakness Tiredness	None known	3.5g
Sodium	Tinned anchovies Table salt Marmite	Dehydration Cramps Low blood pressure	High blood pressure	0.5g
Iron	Egg yolks Sardines Dark green vegetables Offal Beef	Breathlessness Tiredness	Excess rare	8.7g (men) 14.8g (women)
Selenium	Brazil nuts Meat and fish Avocados Lentils	Deficiency is rare	Toxic in excess, it causes foul breath and body odour. Excess would be above 450/day.	50ug

Your Basic Foods

The basic foods on this diet are simple:

1   A daily serving of sugar-free breakfast cereal.

2   Four pieces of fruit per day.

3   Two other servings of carbohydrates, such as bread, yoghurt and pasta.

4   A daily allowance of half a bottle or carton of skimmed milk.

5   Seven grammes of butter every day.

6   One or two portions of an extra-protein food.

Recommended Foods

Cereals

Choose a sugar-free cereal and do not add any sugar, honey or syrup. Try to get used to the taste or add sultanas, dried apricots or dates for natural sweetness. Select from the following cereals:

- Weetabix – two biscuits
- Bran Flakes
- Shredded Wheat – two biscuits
- Special K
- Alpen 'no added sugar' muesli
- Corn Flakes
- Rice Krispies
- Grape Nuts
- Porridge Oats

Bread

Select from the following types of bread:

- White, wholemeal or granary breads
- An average slice should be taken from a medium-sliced loaf
- Uncut bread should weigh 28g per slice

Pasta

All types of pasta are rich in complex carbohydrates. Choose from this list:

- Lasagne
- Penne
- Tagliatelle
- Linguini
- Spaghetti
- Macaroni, etc.

Try to buy the fresh variety of pasta. Each serving is 75g fresh pasta or the equivalent cooked weight of dried pasta.

• • • • • • • • • •

Rice

The following types of rice are recommended:

- Risotto
- Basmati
- Pudding rice
- Long-grain

- *Do not* use dried packet rice with added sauce ingredients

Beans

For sources of carbohydrates in beans, choose from this list:

- Kidney beans
- Baked beans
- Butter beans

- Broad beans
- Flageolet beans
- Aduki beans

Vegetables

From the following types of cooked vegetables eat freely:

- Parnsips
- Carrots
- Peas
- Leeks
- Spinach
- Cabbage
- Brussels sprouts
- Onions
- Kale
- Cauliflower
- Broccoli

- Mangetouts
- French/Runner beans
- Asparagus
- Turnips
- Swede
- Sweet potato
- Aubergine
- Mushrooms
- Courgettes
- Artichokes

Salad Vegetables

Again, you can eat freely from the following selection of salad vegetables:

• • • • • • • • • •

- All types of lettuce
- Spinach
- Beetroot
- Cucumber
- Carrot
- Roquette
- Peppers
- Baby corn

- Tomatoes
- Spring onions
- Chicory
- Celery
- White cabbage
- Red cabbage
- Bean sprouts
- Watercress

Dried Fruits

Here the allowance is 50 grammes a time. Choose from the following:

- Apricots
- Figs
- Prunes

- Sultanas
- Raisins
- Currants

Nuts

Select a 30-gramme serving of any of the following:

- Walnuts
- Almonds
- Peanuts
- Brazils

- Hazelnuts
- Pecans
- Pistachios

Fresh Fruit

Eat four pieces of fresh fruit each day. Choose from the following list:

- Apples
- Oranges
- Bananas
- Strawberries

- Blackberries
- Mango
- Blueberries
- Pawpaw

- Grapes
- Pears
- Pineapple
- Peach
- Raspberries

Dairy Products

Select from the following list:

- Hard cheese – Edam, Cheddar, Cheshire, etc.
- Cottage cheese
- Half-fat crème frâiche – 1 dessertspoonful

Daily allowances

As part of your eating plan, make sure you have the following dairy products each day:

- 284 ml skimmed milk
  and
- 7 grammes butter

Condiments, Sauces and Dressings

The following can all be used freely:

- Mustard
- Soy sauce
- Marmite
- Herbs
- Seasonings
- Stock cubes

However, use the following in moderation:

- Tomato ketchup
- Brown sauce

Use once a day only:

- 1 dessertspoonful French dressing
- 1 dessertspoonful mayonnaise or salad cream

- 30 grammes sugar-free jams and fruit spreads
- 2 dessertspoonfuls fat crème frâiche

Bread – White or Brown?

Bread should play a large part in any diet. It lacks sugar and fat, and has a high complex carbohydrate rating. The best thing about bread is that it's versatile, and these days the stunning array of continental breads, in addition to the standard varieties available, means that it doesn't have to be a boring, tasteless and soggy outer covering for a suspicious filling. A nice wedge of fresh soda bread has always been a mouthwatering accompaniment to warming home-made vegetable soup, while thin French toast is still the best way to eat terrines and fish pâtés.

But should you eat white, brown or wholemeal bread? Since the high-fibre revolution started about twenty years ago it has been unfashionable to eat white bread, yet I have to confess to liking it. In common with many others, I find wholemeal products are too rough for me, but don't let me put you off. High fibre is good, and we all need a healthy dose of roughage every day. However, let me advise you that bran has no nutritional value whatsoever and, in fact, passes straight through the system without stopping, which can give rise to the bloatedness that many people find so uncomfortable. If bran affects you, take your fibre in the form of fruit, vegetables and beans.

Type of bread	Calories per slice (28g)	Fibre	Protein	Fat	Vitamins and minerals
White made with refined flour	64	0.3g	2.1	0.4	Contains twice as much calcium as wholemeal, fortified with niacin, iron and thiamin.

Type of bread	Calories per slice (28g)	Fibre	Protein	Fat	Vitamins and minerals
Brown made from wheat flour with some bran removed. May be coloured with caramel.	61	0.8	2.2	0.5	Similar to white bread.
Wholemeal made with flour containing all the bran.	60	1.6	2.6	0.7	Contains 40 per cent more iron than white bread, and higher levels of vitamin B.
Croissant (per 100g)	328	1.6	8.1	20.3	Similar to white bread.
Naan bread	336	1.9	8.9	12.5	Contains more vitamin E than wholemeal bread and 30 per cent more calcium than white bread.
Pitta bread	265	2.2	9.2	1.2	Similar to white bread.

• • • • • • • • • •

'Can I Just Ask You Something?'

Every day my telephone rings and there is a new client on the other end who has just embarked on the first week of her diet. You may have some (or all) of the same queries, so it's best to deal with them before you get going. These are based on real people's questions.

Do I Really Have To Keep Weighing Everything? It Seems Such A Chore And I Can't Really Be Bothered.

You don't have to do anything. And you don't have to go on this diet. No one is telling you to do anything against your will, but if you're determined to succeed and to get back into those jeans, then you need to take some steps in the right direction. That means weighing food, because it was by *not* weighing it and by guessing portions that you gained weight in the first place. It was by not being bothered and eating whatever took your fancy that you gained weight. I'm not suggesting there's anything wrong with eating whatever you fancy if you're happy, but if you're reading this book you're probably not and it's resulted in a figure that you don't want. So make the effort. It doesn't go on for ever because you'll soon get to know what 50 grammes of cereal looks like and how heavy a serving of pasta is without getting out the scales. Take heart: weighing takes just a few seconds, but being slim and getting back into those clothes is a pleasure which is reinforced every time you look in the mirror.

• • • • • • • • • •

I Am On A Gluten-Free Diet. Can I Follow This Plan?

Yes, simply follow the special gluten-free menu suggestions I've set out (see page 96).

The Fruit Allowance Is Rather Small. I Love Fruit And Eat It By The Barrowful. Why Can't I Have More?

Eating fruit 'by the barrowful' is lovely and healthy, but unfortunately it also contains calories just like anything else! Remember, the idea of this diet is to encourage a more balanced view of food and constant snacking is probably a problem for you. Over the next month you should manage to retrain yourself through restriction, and then you can go back to your barrowfuls of fruit if you still want to – but I'll bet you're unlikely to want to, and will have learned to keep an eye out for those calories.

Am I Allowed To Drink Alcohol On This Diet?

Only on your day off. Alcohol in moderation may not be bad for you, but it weakens your resolve. For the next month try to be strong and look on the diet as a training programme. Many of my clients who cut back on high alcohol consumption for this diet find that they lose the desire for it altogether.

You Don't Allow Diet Colas On This Diet, Or Diet Drinks In General. I Find Them Useful To Curb My Hunger Pangs And They Have No Calories. Why Can't I Have Them?

If you're hungry, your body needs *food*. Remember what I said about cravings and your body trying to talk to you? Hunger is a message. But I do believe for good weight maintenance that you should stick to mealtimes and scheduled food breaks. After you've retrained yourself, the hunger pangs will stop, but in the meantime, don't dampen them with fizzy drinks; have pure water instead. Most diet drinks contain caffeine, which is addictive

• • • • • • • • • •

and bad for you, and they also contain high levels of artificial sweeteners which only encourage your sweet tooth. Stay away from them. Wait for your meal, drink water, and your food will taste all the better because you have looked forward to it.

Why No Diet Yoghurts Or Desserts?

Most of them still contain sugar or other additives which can cause bloating and flatulence. They are also pumped full of air so you seem to be getting more than there really is, and at the end of the day they can be unsatisfying. It is far better to have pure, unadulterated live yoghurt with fresh or dried fruit to give you that bit of sweetness which you are used to after a meal.

I Just Want To Get My Stomach Smaller – The Rest Of Me Is Fine. How Can This Diet Help Me?

You need to read my book, *5 Days to a Flatter Stomach* (Boxtree), which has a similar diet but concentrates on the other causes of a big stomach, such as bloating. For example, you're allowed fruit, but only in the evenings. You're allowed vegetables, but not pulses, broccoli or sprouts. And you can only eat white bread. That diet will also help you because its main theme is frequent eating and this has been proved to be an important factor in getting your stomach flat.

Will This Diet Help Me To Reduce Fat On My Thighs?

The whole plan, including the exercise, will help, yes. No diet can target thighs or any other part of your body, but if you carry your excess fat on your thighs, it's likely that this is where it will go from. I think you'll have spectacular results.

• • • • • • • • • •

I Am Semi-Disabled And Have Arthritis In Both Knees. I Can't Exercise Much, But I Am Desperate To Lose Weight As I Am 16 stone-plus. Will This Diet Work For Me?

Yes, it will. I've included one special menu for arthritis sufferers which should help your condition (see page 99), and you should do any exercise you can. In addition to this, I've given you some general guidelines about diet and six days of meals. After that, you'll probably be able to devise your own meals for the next three weeks. This diet will help you to reduce inflammation and lose weight, which is important for easing the stress on your joints.

I Lead A Hectic Life As A Community Nurse And Often Have To Take Meal Breaks In My Car. How Can I Possibly Fit This Diet Into My Lifestyle?

You still have to eat! I have included 'snacker's' menus which divide up the basic foods for you into five or six small snacks (see pages 92–4). The secret lies in the planning and what you must avoid at all costs is going for hours on end without eating too much in the evening. As long as you plan ahead and prepare food when it's convenient to do so, such as on a Sunday, you should have a fridge stocked and ready for you to devise a week's home-made diet snacks.

I Go Out To Eat A Lot As The Job I Do Involves A Lot Of Socializing For Business. How Can I Stick To A Diet When I Have To Eat Restaurant Food?

There's nothing special about restaurant food! Most menus have plain fish or meat, salads and vegetables, and they're the best to go for. A word of advice: don't go for risottos or pasta dishes when you are out as I have seen the amount of butter and oils that can be poured over them, and ask if the restaurant adds butter to their vegetables before serving. If they

• • • • • • • • • •

do, ask them not to. Ask for sauces to be left off meat or fish, too.

It's bad manners to go without a course when everyone else is having one, so always choose something and then pick at it. If there isn't a fruit option for pudding and everyone is having one, choose anything – it doesn't matter what – and have half of it. It won't break your calorie bank.

I'm Not Used To This Kind Of Diet And I Feel Out Of Control. I'm Not Sure That I Want To Be Told What To Eat

You have two options: to stay as you are or to go forward. No one is forcing you into either choice, but please understand: you weren't in control before, which is why you have this problem. Your appetite was controlling you. Now you truly are in the driving seat because you are strong enough to resist temptation. The process is a bit hard at first because you are breaking yourself of old habits. But very soon you will have the eating habits of a slim person and you will emerge 'reinvented'.

Your Personal Measurement Record

First of all, you need to know where you're starting from. You should weigh and measure yourself so that you can monitor where the weight is going from, or which bits are being toned up. Write down your current clothes size too. When you have filled in your details, don't check them again for two weeks. In a month's time you will be able to compare your first and last charts, and hopefully you'll have a wonderful surprise!

The reason for measuring the area just underneath the bustline is because weight is often stored on – and lost from – your back. Therefore, the general bust measurement can be

• • • • • • • • • •

mistaken for breast size when it incorporates your back and weight loss that registers on scales often can't be seen. 'I've lost weight – but I don't know where from!' is a common cry from my clients. Only by exercising and toning will you be sure that the stubborn areas of fat that stop you from getting back into those jeans are slimmed down.

Keep this record to remind you where you lost the weight.

Personal Measurement Record

Date ....

Weight .... kg

Bust .... cm

Chest (men) .... cm

Under bust (ribcage) .... cm

Waist .... cm

Pelvis (hip bones) .... cm

Hips .... cm

Top of the thigh .... cm

Above the knee .... cm

Dress size .... cm

• • • • • • • • • •

After Two Weeks

Weight .... kg

Bust .... cm

Chest (men) .... cm

Under bust (ribcage) .... cm

Waist .... cm

Pelvis (hip bones) .... cm

Hips .... cm

Top of the thigh .... cm

Above the knee .... cm

Dress size .... cm

At the End of the Month

Weight .... kg

Bust .... cm

Chest (men) .... cm

Under bust (ribcage) .... cm

Waist .... cm

Pelvis (hip bones) .... cm

Hips .... cm

Top of the thigh .... cm

Above the knee .... cm

Dress size .... cm

• • • • • • • • • •

Menus for a Month

Here are your weekly menu plans for the next month. You start with a list of proteins from which you can choose every day – these are your meal 'bases' – and you then have a different list of carbohydrate foods for each week. Every week I have devised a programme of 'standard' menu suggestions for you – with and without meat – but you can devise your own if you have special considerations to take into account. These follow afterwards – you can use these every week, if you like. In fact, all the suggested menu plans have been designed so that you can mix and match any four weeks – but don't mix and match the menus per day. They have been devised to work best in a six-day sequence. All the recipes are in the back of the book (see pages 138–78).

Remember:

- Drink plain water with your meals and have as much tea and decaffeinated coffee as you like.
- Alcohol should only be drunk on your day 'off' the diet.
- Keep your food diary religiously. Although it seems a fiddle, it's worth it. It takes just a few seconds to write down what you've eaten. Don't cheat: remember, you can fool anybody but yourself, so if you eat it – *write it down!*
- Check your calories all the time by looking at the calorie counter at the back of the book (see pages 131–7).

● ● ● ● ● ● ● ● ● ●

Keeping a Food Diary

Whenever a new client comes to me, their first task is to keep a food diary for a week, which I can then analyse. They mustn't try to impress me or to hide anything, and they write down everything that passes their lips during those seven days, even if it is a lick of the spoon whilst making a cake! This gives me an idea of their eating habits as well as what they are actually eating. Then, when I have given them their personal diet, they continue to keep a record, and you will be keeping the same sort of diary for yourself.

It may seem tedious, but after a month the diary isn't necessary. You can go back to it whenever problems arise because it's a good way to spot extra calories. You don't have to become a calorie fanatic. Instead, you simply develop a sixth sense about your food and the calories you are burning, and that is what people mean when they say 'I'm just careful'.

Why Bother?

You try to watch your eating for three reasons:

1   You can see the calories you consume through tasting, nibbling and picking at food.
2   You realize the calorie content of 'good' foods such as salads, fruit and vegetables, which can still mount up.
3   It allows you to be in control and to decide just how you want to distribute your calories during each day. This means that you can save calories for special occasions and still not gain weight.

How to Keep the Diary

Leave your diary in the kitchen, car or office desk – wherever it will be most handy for you. I have written a sample page (see below) and after you've entered your personal calorie allowance you simply deduct calories as you go along. Start with the foods that you know you are going to have, such as your milk allowance, cereal and so on, then you'll know how many calories you have left for the rest of the day.

Deducting calories is a more efficient and successful way of monitoring your food intake than adding them up. You only have to keep this diary for the next month, so stick with it! You're going to be lighter, more shapely and slimmer – *and* you're going to get back into those jeans!

• • • • • • • • • •

Your Daily Record

If you decide to choose your own meals each day, it is important that you keep a record of your calories. Here is an example of how the record should be kept:

Day One: Date

Food Eaten	Starting Calorie Allowance 1,400
(Less milk and butter allowance)	146
	1,254
Less cereal, grapefruit	235
	1,019
Less tuna sandwich, salad and an apple	352
	667
Less fruit teacake	230
	437
Less roast chicken, vegetables and mango sorbet	440
Total	− 3 calories

You would have almost broken even on your calorie allowance that day. Therefore, the message is to keep a careful track of everything that passes your lips!

• • • • • • • • •

Protein Foods – Your Daily Allowance

Choose *one* or *two* foods only per day from this list and adjust your intake from other sources of calories accordingly.

Type of Food	Calories	Day: 1	2	3	4	5	6	7
30g nuts	180							
175g chicken	300							
125g red meat	200							
150g Quorn	144							
150g Tofu	100							
100g smoked salmon	160							
150g fresh salmon	318							
100g sardines	184							
100g tuna fish	112							
100g prawns	110							
150g white fish	168							
30g hard cheese	120							
100g cottage cheese	120							
1 egg	90							

Carbohydrates – Week One Allowance

Choose *seven* portions of carbohydrates each day. Do not choose any food twice. Tick the boxes to remind yourself that you have eaten them.

Type of Food	Calories	Day: 1 2 3 4 5 6 7

Choose three of the following foods each day:

Type of Food	Calories
40g cereal	158
3 slices bread	240
2 slices bread	160
150g potatoes	150
225g potatoes	250
125g sweetcorn	125
125g baked beans	125
1 small carton plain yoghurt	88
1 slice Bran Cake (see page 144)	176

Choose four of the following foods each day:

Type of Food	Calories
1 banana	90
150g strawberries	48
Small bunch grapes	90
1 mango, cubed	110
1 apple	55
1 pear	45

Week One: Menu Planner

Day	Total Proteins Consumed	Total Carbohydrates Consumed	Total Calorie Allowance Used
1			
2			
3			
4			
5			
6			
7			

Total calories used in Week One:

_____

* Allow yourself one 'day off' on each menu planner.

Week One – Suggested Standard Menus

For recipes accompanied by an asterisk, see Recipes for Success (pages 138–78).

Breakfast Cereal Sliced banana	**Breakfast** Half a portion of Fresh Fruit Salad*	**Breakfast** Cereal One slice toast
Lunch Salad sandwich Apple	**Lunch** Egg & cress sandwich Yoghurt	**Lunch** Large jacket potato Salad Yoghurt
Snack Grapes	**Snack** Cereal & milk	**Snack** Mango cubes

Main Meal
Roast chicken
Boiled potatoes
Steamed vegetables
Poached pear*
	Main Meal
	Lamb chop
	Small jacket potato
	Steamed vegetables
	Half portion of Fresh Fruit
	   Salad*
		Main Meal
		Sardines on two slices
		   toast
		Pear & Apple Charlotte*

1,304 calories	1,222 calories	1,356 calories
Breakfast Cereal	**Breakfast** Strawberries & yoghurt	**Breakfast** Yoghurt with 15g flaked almonds Half a sliced apple

Lunch
Cottage cheese & Fresh
   Fruit Salad*
	Lunch
	Home-made Fresh
	   Vegetable Soup*
	Two slices bread
		Lunch
		Two slices smoked salmon
		Two slices bread
		Apple & Grape Salad

Snack Slice Bran Cake*	**Snack** Banana	**Snack** Pear
Main Meal Poached Fillet of Salmon Mashed potatoes Mixed salad Mango cubes	**Main Meal** Shepherd's Pie Peas/carrots Baked apple	**Main Meal** Vegetable Stir-fry with Sweetcorn Baked Banana*
1,438 calories	1,217 calories	1,033 calories

• • • • • • • • • •

Week One – Suggested Vegetarian Menus

These menus include some fish and dairy produce. For recipes accompanied by an asterisk, see Recipes for Success (pages 138–78).

Breakfast Cereal One slice toast	**Breakfast** Sliced mango and banana	**Breakfast** Two slices toast Sugar-free marmalade
Lunch Salad sandwich Yoghurt Pear	**Lunch** Bombay Potato Salad* Pear	**Lunch** Jacket potato Mixed salad Mango, strawberry & grape salad
Snack Strawberries & grapes	**Snack** Cereal with sliced apple	**Snack** Apple
Main Meal Quorn & Pepper Kebabs* Roasted Vegetables Slice Bran Cake*	**Main Meal** Beans on two slices toast Grapes	**Main Meal** Red Bean and Tomato Curry*
1,284 calories	1,239 calories	1,264 calories
Breakfast Cereal Fresh Fruit Salad* Pear, apple & grapes	**Breakfast** Baked beans on one slice toast Grapes	**Breakfast** Cereal
Lunch Cottage Cheese & Grape Sandwich	**Lunch** 'Covent Garden' Asparagus or Watercress Soup One slice bread Strawberries & yoghurt	**Lunch** Cheese salad with walnuts Strawberries
No snack	**Snack** Banana & apple	**Snack** Salad sandwich Apple, grapes
Main Meal Jacket potato with tuna fish Mixed salad Mango Sorbet*	**Main Meal** Grilled cod Mashed potato Puréed carrots	**Main Meal** Curried Vegetables with Cashew Nuts
1,146 calories	1,106 calories	1,215 calories

• • • • • • • • •

Carbohydrates – Week Two Allowance

Choose *seven* portions of carbohydrates each day of Week Two. Do not choose any food twice. Tick the boxes to remind yourself that you have eaten them.

Type of Food	Calories	Day: 1 2 3 4 5 6 7

Choose three of the following foods each day:

2 slices bread	160	
40g cereal	158	
100g long-grain rice (cooked)	170	
30g pudding rice (dry weight)	102	
30g semolina or sago	95	
568 ml milk (extra)	190	
2 slices crispbread	56	
30g dried fruit	78	
125g lentils or beans	125	

Choose four of the following foods each day:

284 ml fresh orange juice	57	
150g fresh pineapple	45	
1 apple (baking or eating)	55	
1 orange	40	
1 peach	45	
1 pawpaw	55	
150g plums (without sugar)	43	
1 banana	90	

Week Two: Menu Planner

Day	Total Proteins Consumed	Total Carbohydrates Consumed	Total Calorie Allowance Used
1			
2			
3			
4			
5			
6			
7			

Total calories used in Week Two:

_____

* Allow yourself one 'day off'.

• • • • • • • • •

Week Two – Suggested Standard Menus

For recipes accompanied by an asterisk, see Recipes for Success (pages 138–78).

Breakfast 284ml fresh orange juice Two slices toast Sugar-free jam	**Breakfast** Cereal Tea or coffee	**Breakfast** Boiled egg One slice toast Tea or coffee Glass fresh orange juice
Lunch Cheese salad Eating apple Peach	**Lunch** Open prawn sandwich Apple	**Lunch** Mixed Fresh Fruit Salad* made from three pieces fruit
Snack Two slices crispbread, sugar-free jam or Marmite Butter from allowance	**Snack** Handful dried apricots or sultanas Peach	**No snack**
Main Meal Chicken Curry with Rice Fresh pineapple	**Main Meal** Stir-fry Chicken on Carrot & Orange Salad* Stewed plums	**Main Meal** Chilli Con Carne with Kidney Beans & Rice*
1,102 calories	1,112 calories	973 calories

Breakfast	**Breakfast** Fresh orange juice Cereal Boiled egg	**Breakfast** Two slices crispbread with sugar-free jam Orange juice
Lunch Salad sandwich Orange, peach	**Lunch** Lentil soup Two slices bread	**Lunch** Cottage Cheese Salad Rice Pudding
Snack Cereal with pineapple	**Snack** Apple	**Snack** Apple & peach
Main Meal Beef Casserole Mixed vegetables Baked apple with sultanas	**Main Meal** Chicken Casserole or Chicken Stir-fry & Vegetables Pineapple & peach mixed	**Main Meal** Lamb chop Mixed vegetables Roast Pineapple*
1,067 calories	1,079 calories	1,000 calories

• • • • • • • • •

Week Two – Suggested Vegetarian Menus

These menus include some fish and dairy produce. For recipes accompanied by an asterisk, see Recipes for Success (pages 138–78).

Breakfast Fresh orange juice Cereal	**Breakfast** Mixed Fruit Salad	**Breakfast** Two slices toast Poached egg Glass fresh orange juice
Lunch Feta & Walnut Salad* Apple	**Lunch** Mixed Bean Salad with Quorn Glass fresh orange juice	**Lunch** Tuna & Rice Salad Apple
Snack Two slices crispbread Cottage cheese Peach	**Snack** Cereal Glass milk	**Snack** Banana milk shake
Main Meal Vegetable curry Hot spiced oranges*	**Main Meal** Cauliflower Cheese Sliced tomatoes	**Main Meal** Steamed Haddock with Plain Boiled Vegetables Poached Peach*
1,075 calories	988 calories	1,233 calories

Breakfast Cereal Two slices toast	**Breakfast** Cereal	**Breakfast** Two slices crispbread Fresh orange juice

Lunch
Peach
Handful peanuts
Banana
	Lunch
	Sweet & Sour Vegetables
	    with Rice
	Peach
		Lunch
		Cottage cheese & Fresh
		    Fruit Salad*

Snack Two slices crispbread & Marmite Fresh orange juice	**Snack** Handful sultanas Salad sandwich Orange	**Snack** Banana

Main Meal
Winter Salad* with Grated
    Apple
	Main Meal
	Quorn and Pepper Kebabs*
	    with Sliced Pawpaw &
	    Pineapple
		Main Meal
		Spiced Vegetable Risotto
		    with Green Lentils*

892 calories	1,107 calories	878 calories

• • • • • • • • • •

Carbohydrates: Week Three Allowance

Type of Food	Calories	Day: 1 2 3 4 5 6 7

Choose three of the following foods each day:

2 slices bread	160
150g (cooked weight) pasta	180
150g noodles (cooked)	108
50g couscous	187
40g oats	107
30g dates	78
125g sweetcorn	125
1 jacket potato (200g)	200

Choose four of the following foods each day:

200g stewed apple	80
Small bunch grapes	90
½ avocado pear	130
100g blueberries	64
½ grapefruit	47
200g stewed rhubarb	64
150g tinned peaches (no sugar)	60
1 apple	55
150g gooseberries (no sugar)	35
1 pear	45

Week Three: Menu Planner

Day	Total Proteins Consumed	Total Carbohydrates Consumed	Total Calorie Allowance Used
1			
2			
3			
4			
5			
6			
7			

Total calories used in Week Three:

_____

* Allow yourself one 'day off'.

• • • • • • • • •

Week Three – Suggested Standard Menus

For recipes accompanied by an asterisk, see Recipes for Success (pages 138–78).

Breakfast Porridge	**Breakfast** Two slices toast	**Breakfast** Boiled egg Two slices toast

Lunch
Tuna Salad with
  Sweetcorn
Grapes
	Lunch
	½ Avocado with Prawns
	Grapes
		Lunch
		Roasted Vegetables &
		  Couscous Salad
		Apple

Snack Handful nuts	**Snack** Grapes, apple	**No snack**

Main Meal
Vegetable Lasagne
Tinned peaches &
  blueberries
	Main Meal
	Spaghetti Bolognese
	Mixed Salad with
	  Sweetcorn
	Stewed Rhubarb
		Main Meal
		Macaroni Cheese
		Three-Fruit Salad

1,167 calories	1,372 calories	1,138 calories

Breakfast ½ grapefruit	**Breakfast** Porridge with Chopped Dates	**Breakfast** ½ grapefruit One slice toast
Lunch Cheese salad Apple	**Lunch** Pasta Twists with Pesto & Nut Dressing*	**Lunch** Tomato Soup One slice bread Apple
Snack Salad sandwich Dates Grapes	**No snack**	**Snack** Bowl porridge Chopped dates

Main Meal
Chicken Stir-fry with
  Noodles
Tinned peaches
	Main Meal
	Smoked Salmon & Avocado
	  Salad*
	Apple, Blueberry & Grape
	  Salad
		Main Meal
		Roast Chicken
		Steamed Vegetables
		Stewed Rhubarb

1,259 calories	1,233 calories	1,115 calories

• • • • • • • • • •

Week Three – Suggested Vegetarian Menus

These menus include some fish and dairy products.

Breakfast ½ grapefruit Scrambled egg One slice toast	Breakfast Porridge	Breakfast Two slices toast ½ grapefruit
Lunch Roast Vegetables with Couscous Apple	**Lunch** Cold Salmon with Pasta Twists Apple & grapes mixed	**Lunch** Macaroni Cheese with Tomatoes Tinned peaches
Snack One slice toast Grapes	**Snack** Salad sandwich Stewed Rhubarb	**No snack**
Main Meal Cannelloni Stuffed with Spinach & Almonds* Stewed apple	**Main Meal** Quorn & Pepper Kebabs* Tinned peaches	**Main Meal** Egg Mayonnaise with Sweetcorn Apple & grapes mixed
1,295 calories	1,397 calories	1,127 calories

Breakfast Porridge ½ grapefruit	Breakfast Porridge Tinned peaches	Breakfast One slice toast Boiled egg ½ grapefruit
Lunch Spicy Vegetable Salad Stir-Fry with Sweetcorn	**Lunch** Waldorf Salad	**Lunch** Welsh Rarebit One slice toast
No snack	**Snack** Two slices toast & Marmite	**Snack** Bowl porridge Apple & grapes mixed
Main Meal Lasagne Verdi* Spinach & Avocado Salad* Apple & blueberries	**Main Meal** Salmon Stir-fry with Noodles Stewed Apple	**Main Meal** Vegetable Bolognese with Spaghetti Tinned peaches
1,012 calories	1,347 calories	1,118 calories

• • • • • • • • • •

Carbohydrates: Week Four Allowance

Type of Food	Calories	Day: 1 2 3 4 5 6 7

Choose three of the following foods each day:

Type of Food	Calories	
40g sugar-free cereal	130	
2 slices olive/tomato bread	160	
1 baguette (75g)	210	
1 pitta pocket	170	
Naan bread (any type)	370	
Croissant	230	
3 slices wholemeal bread	160	
2 slices multigrain crispbread	56	
150g potatoes	150	
Fruit teacake	230	
1 carton live yoghurt	88	

Choose four of the following foods each day:

Type of Food	Calories	
150g raspberries	54	
100g prunes in fruit juice	88	
100g grapefruit segments	95	
1 apple	55	
1 banana	90	
1 slice melon	45	
20 grapes	60	

Week Four: Menu Planner

Day	Total Proteins Consumed	Total Carbohydrates Consumed	Total Calorie Allowance Used
1			
2			
3			
4			
5			
6			
7			

Total calories used in Week Four:

_____

* Allow yourself one 'day off'.

• • • • • • • • •

Week Four – Suggested Standard Menus

For recipes accompanied by an asterisk, see Recipes for Success (pages 138–78).

Breakfast Cereal	**Breakfast** Two slices wholemeal toast Grapefruit segments	**Breakfast** Prunes in juice mixed with grapefruit segments Croissant Sugar-free jam
Lunch ½ melon filled with raspberries	**Lunch** Baguette filled with tuna and salad Apple	**Lunch** Teacake Banana
Snack Two slices crispbread with Marmite Apple	**Snack** One slice toast Marmite Banana	**No snack**
Main Meal Chicken Curry with Garlic Naan bread Baked Banana*	**Main Meal** Jacket potato Cheese Mixed Salad Raspberry Sorbet*	**Main Meal** Roast beef or lamb Boiled potatoes Cauliflower Carrots, peas Baked Apple
1,362 calories	1,372 calories	1,394 calories

Breakfast Croissant Sugar-free jam	**Breakfast** Cereal Grapefruit	**Breakfast** Prunes Two slices crispbread with Marmite
Lunch Pitta Pocket with Tuna & Salad	**Lunch** Chicken sandwich Apple	**Lunch** Melon Balls with Prawns & Dressing
Snack Apple & banana	**Snack** Two slices crispbread with Marmite Prunes	**Snack** Fruit teacake
Main Meal Jacket potato Winter Salad* Melon & raspberries	**Main Meal** Poached egg on one slice wholemeal toast Baked Banana*	**Main Meal** Italian Chicken with Tomato & Basil Sauce Two slices Olive Bread Salad Raspberry & Banana Mousse
1,142 calories	1,200 calories	1,394 calories

Week Four – Suggested Vegetarian Menus

These menus include some fish and dairy products.

Breakfast Yoghurt with prunes	**Breakfast** Cereal & grapefruit	**Breakfast** Cereal
Lunch Baguette filled with Roasted Vegetables Apple	**Lunch** Cheese on two slices wholemeal toast Banana	**Lunch** Tomato soup Tomato bread Grapes
Snack Pitta pocket & salad	**Snack** Grapes	**No snack**
Main Meal Jacket potato filled with Vegetable Chilli Melon & raspberries	**Main Meal** Smoked Salmon on Potato Cakes with Crème Fraîche* Carton yoghurt and sliced apple	**Main Meal** Italian baguette halved, topped with tomatoes, cheese, olives, anchovies & oregano Three-fruit Salad
991 calories	1,434 calories	1,194 calories
Breakfast Croissant with sugar-free jam Grapefruit segments	**Breakfast** Scrambled egg on one slice toast	**Breakfast** Cereal One slice toast
Lunch Wholemeal bread salad sandwich Apple	**Lunch** Tomatoes on two slices toast Slice melon	**Lunch** Jacket potato with Winter Salad* Grapefruit segments
Snack Banana & grapes	**Snack** Teacake Apple & grapes	**Snack** Feta cheese & walnut sandwich Grapes
Main Meal Baked Brie Ciabatta*	**Main Meal** Cod & Prawn Pie with Mashed Potato Topping Green vegetables Baked Banana*	**Main Meal** Courgette & Tomato Gratin* Melon & raspberries
1,256 calories	1,428 calories	1,323 calories

The Exercises

Your Waist – the Forgotten Bit in the Middle

1. Take up the position as shown. Make sure the small of your back is pressed downwards on to the mat or carpet

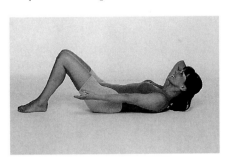

and that your pelvis is tilted upwards towards your navel. Place your right hand under your head (not on your neck), and look up at the ceiling. Breathe in.

2. Breathe out and reach sideways to your left foot. Make sure that your right elbow is not facing the celing. This is a sideways 'swivel'. You don't need to touch your foot – making the effort and the correct movement is enough to

have the right effect. Do twelve reaches on this side, rest for twenty seconds, then change hands and repeat on the other side.

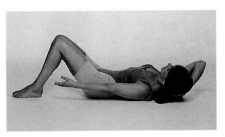

• **Your Goal:** a total of twenty-four repetitions on each side.

It's My Stomach!

1. Take up the position as shown. Keep your knees together at all times. This is important because during the effort of 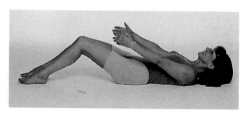 abdominal exercises, the body tries to help itself by transferring the effort anywhere else it can, and that means the powerful muscles in your thighs, the quadriceps muscles. Holding your knees together renders your legs inactive. Press back downwards, breathe in and then breathe out. Cradle your head in one hand as before – don't pull on your neck – and raise your head and shoulders off the floor if you need to.

2. *Stay there* and breathe easily. Now, release your hand, reach forwards with 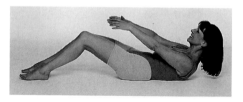 both hands as shown, tuck your pelvis up, press your stomach downards and *hold* the position.

3. 'Pulse' six times. *Hold.* Breathe in and then breathe out.

4. Bring your fingertips back to your temples and *slowly* release back on to the floor.

• **Your Goal:** Do six repetitions, rest and then do six again.

• • • • • • • • • •

It's This Bit on My Hips

1. Sit cross-legged on the floor, as shown. Place your right hand on the floor and raise your left hand above your head.

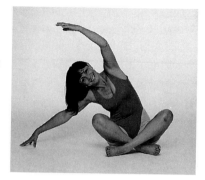

2. Let the fingertips of your right hand slide slowly along the floor, a couple of centimetres at a time. *Hold* after every few centimetres. Breathe in and then breathe out, and let your top arm *stretch* over the top of your head. Keep both buttocks planted firmly on the floor and *hold* again. You should feel a strong stretch right down your side and into your hip. Slowly come back to the centre using your right hand to 'walk' you back to the upright. Release your top arm and repeat on your other side.

• **Your Goal:** Do three repetitions on each side, rest and then repeat. Always do this exercise at the end of your aerobic workout.

Beating Those Saddlebags

1. Stand upright with your feet together. Take a side step and bring the other leg behind, as shown. It looks a bit like a curtsey.

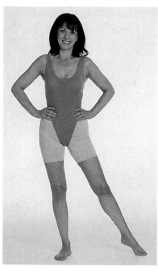

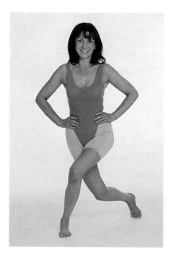

2. Step your feet back together again and repeat on the other side. You can keep your hands on your hips or use them for balance as in the picture. As you curtsey, bring your hands to your thighs for balance. The movement is *step – curstey – step back together – curtsey* on the other side, and so on.

• **Your Goal:** Do twelve repetitions on each side, rest and then repeat if possible. Stretch out afterwards, as shown in stretch 1.

• • • • • • • • • •

Inner Thighs

1. To shape up
   your thighs,
   lie on floor,
   as shown,
   with your top
   leg over your
   bottom leg.
   Now, breathe
   in.

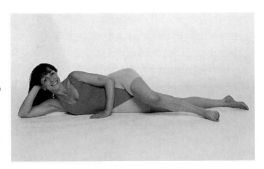

2. Breathe out
   while you
   slowly raise
   your lower
   leg and *hold*.
   Try to breathe
   easily and
   don't raise
   your leg too

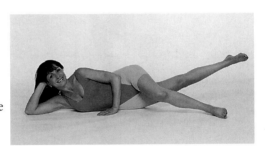

high. Now *stretch* your toes and point them, feeling your lower leg elongating and going further. *Hold* for five seconds and then release to the floor. (The pace of this exercise should be about six a minute.)

• **Your Goal:** Do ten repetitions with each leg, rest and then repeat. Stretch out, as shown in stretch 2.

Crouching Quadricep Pliés

1. With feet slightly wider than hip distance apart, bend your knees and place your forearms on the back of a chair, as shown. Lower your hips until your knees are at right angles to the floor.

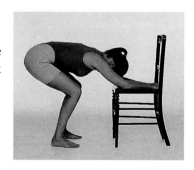

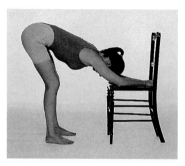

2. Raise your bottom 15–20cm, then lower again, keeping your shoulders down by the chair. This must be done slowly, raising to a count of four, and then releasing to a count of four.

• **Your Goal:** Do twelve repetitions, rest and repeat – it's hard!

Declining Hamstring Bridges

1. Lie on the floor with your feet on a chair use both feet to start with.

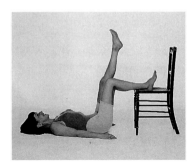

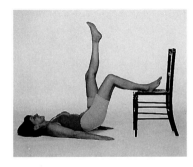

2. Slowly raise your buttocks off the floor making sure that you don't thrust your hips towards the ceiling, which would simply flex your stomach muscles. Do sixteen of these.

3. In the advanced move, place one foot on your opposite thigh, or extend the leg into the air, as shown.

• **Your Goal:** Do sixteen repetitions with both feet on the chair, then twelve for each single leg. Rest and repeat.

• • • • • • • • •

Glute Sweeps

1. Take up the position, as shown, on your elbows and knees. Keep your hips square to the floor. Raise your right leg, making sure your knee is facing towards the floor and not turning outwards. Do not dip your back and keep your stomach pulled in tightly.

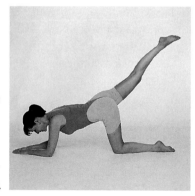

2. Slowly lower your right leg *crossing it over* the left leg and touching your toe to the floor. Raise it again slowly and make sure you squeeze your buttock tightly as you hold your leg at its highest point. Do twelve of these, rest and then change legs and repeat.

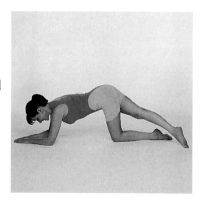

• **Your Goal:** Do twelve repetitions on each leg, rest and repeat.

Standing Dips

1. Take up the position, as shown, with one leg behind the other, then take a small step to the side for balance. Lean forwards, feeling all the effort in your front buttock. Dip downwards and raise yourself again, eight times. Change legs and repeat.

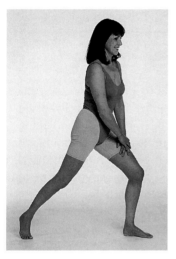 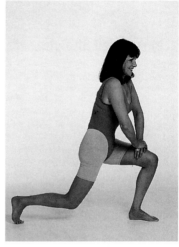

• **Your Goal:** Do eight repetitions on each leg, rest and repeat. After two weeks you should increase this to three sets on each leg.

• • • • • • • • • •

1. Outer Thigh Stretch

Sit on floor, cross-legged, and inhale. Exhale, and slowly lean foward over your legs as shown, placing your hands on the floor and lowering your head. Hold for 10 seconds.

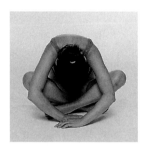

2. Inner Thigh Stretch

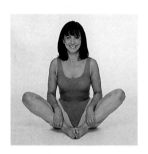

Sit on floor with the soles of your feet together. Place your hands on your ankles, breathe in and lift your ribcage. Slightly lean fowards, pressing your knees downwards to the floor, feeling the stretch in your inner thighs. Hold for a count of 10, release and repeat the stretch.

3. Quadriceps Stretch

Stand sideways to a chair, maintaning balance with one hand. Bring a foot backwards towards your buttocks and hold. Make sure your knees are touching, your supporting leg is slightly 'soft' at the knee, and your back is not arched. Hold for a count of 20. Change legs.

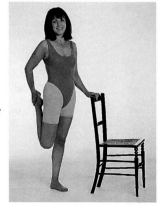

• • • • • • • • • •

4. Hamstring Stretch

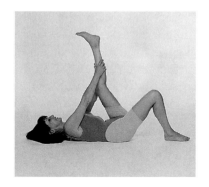

Lie on the floor as shown, one foot flat. Lift the other leg and stretch to the ceiling as much or as little as you can. Hold behind the calf or thigh. Try not to lift your buttocks off the floor. Hold for a count of 20, change legs.

5. Gluteal Stretch

Lie on the floor as shown, one foot flat. Rest your arms and hands on the floor by your sides. Place your left foot across the opposite knee and lift your right foot from the floor until you feel a stretch in your buttock. Hold for 20 seconds, change legs.

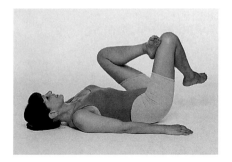

6. Waist Stretch

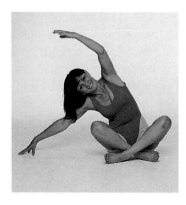

Sit cross-legged on the floor. Raise both hands above your head. Breathe in. Keep your right arm high, breathe out and slowly lower your left arm until your fingertips touch the floor. Hold and slowly 'walk' your fingertips away until the stretch is strong. Hold for a count of 10, slowly return to the centre and relax. Repeat on the other side.

7. Abdominal Stretch

Lie on your stomach with forearms flat on the floor. Breathe in, then breathe out as you slowly press backwards until you feel a stretch in your abdomen. Keep your neck in line with your back, hold for 20 seconds, release and repeat.

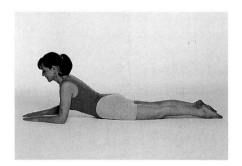

• • • • • • • • •

More Menu Ideas

The meat and non-meat menus plans I've suggested for every week may not suit your tastes, needs or budget. So on the following pages you'll find a few 'special' programmes, which you can substitute for any of the previous weekly plans – or indeed, repeat every week. Just don't mix and match the days!

Suggested 'Gourmet' Menus

These are finer meals created from simple ingredients.

Breakfast Fruit salad of apples, grapes, strawberries	**Breakfast** Cereal Two slices toast	**Breakfast** Cereal Banana
Lunch Smoked Salmon on Potato Cakes* Green salad	**Lunch** Strawberry & Cucumber Salad*	**Lunch** Salmon Mousseline* French toast Grapes
Snack One pear One banana	**Snack** Slice Bran Cake* Apple	**Snack** Pear & yoghurt
Main Meal Fillet steak Mixed salad Sweetcorn	**Main Meal** Poached Cod* Dauphinoise potatoes Mango Sorbet*	**Main Meal** Lamb Kebab Mixed Peppers Green Salad Strawberry Sorbet*
1,279 calories	1,191 calories	1,299 calories
Breakfast One scrambled egg Two slices toast	**Breakfast** Mushrooms on toast	**Breakfast** Cereal
Lunch Two-Pear Salad* Strawberries Yoghurt	**Lunch** Salade Niçoise* Slice Bran Cake	**Lunch** Vichyssoise Soup Two slices bread Pear
Snack Cereal, apple	**Snack** Banana, Grape & Apple Salad	**Snack** Yoghurt
Main Meal Warm Chicken Salad* Baked Banana*	**Main Meal** Szechuan Pepper & Tofu Stir-fry* Caramelized Pear*	**Main Meal** Roast Fillet Salmon Boiled New Potatoes Mangetout or Green Salad Mango & Banana Kebabs
1,148 calories	1,394 calories	1,203 calories

Suggested 'Spicy' Menus

Breakfast Toasted teacake Grapefruit	**Breakfast** Cereal Banana	**Breakfast** Prunes Two slices wholemeal toast

Lunch
Bombay Potato Salad* with
  mixed peppers
	Lunch
	Two slices crispbread
	Cottage cheese
	Grapes
		Lunch
		Baguette pizza topped with
		  tomatoes, olives, cheese
		  & oregano
		Apple

Snack Apple & banana	**Snack** Apple	**No snack**

Main Meal
Vegetable chilli with sun-
  dried tomato bread
Raspberries
	Main Meal
	Spicy Yoghurt-baked
	  chicken
	Garlic potatoes
	Broccoli
		Main Meal
		Jacket potato with chilli con
		  carne filling
		Mixed salad
		Melon & ginger with
		  raspberries

1,128 calories	1,153 calories	1,185 calories

Breakfast Prunes & grapefruit One slice toast	**Breakfast** Two slices toast Sugar-free jam	**Breakfast** Apple, banana & grapes Croissant

Lunch
Chicken Tikka
Sandwich
Apple
	Lunch
	Pitta pocket filled with
	  vegetable chilli
	Grapes
		Lunch
		Baguette filled with curried
		  tuna & salad

Snack Two slices crispbread Marmite	**Snack** Cereal	**No snack**

Main Meal
Baby Balti vegetables
Naan bread
Grapes
	Main Meal
	Beef in red wine with Red
	  Peppers, Onions &
	  Paprika
	Broccoli, cauliflower
	Three-fruit Salad
		Main Meal
		Lamb Curry
		Bombay Potato Salad
		Mixed vegetables
		Raspberry Sorbet*

1,510 calories	1,286 calories	1,347 calories

• • • • • • • • •

Suggested 'Snacker's' Menu: Plan One

These ideas have been designed for people with erratic lives.

Breakfast Slice toast Marmite	**Breakfast** Baked beans on toast	**Breakfast** Slice toast Sugar-free spread
Snack Cheese sandwich Apple	**Snack** Banana sandwich	**Snack** Apple, banana
Late Lunch Slice Bran Cake* Banana	**Late Lunch** Jacket potato with tuna	**No late Lunch**
Main Meal Roast chicken Steamed vegetables Boiled potatoes	**Main Meal** Large colourful salad with sweetcorn	**Main Meal** Cheese on two slices toast
Snack Cereal	**Snack** Carton yoghurt with apple	**Snack** Mixed salad with sweetcorn
Snack Grapes	**No snack**	**Snack** Fruit salad with mangoes, grapes & strawberries
1,298 calories	1,176 calories	1,094 calories

No Breakfast	**No Breakfast**	**No Breakfast**
Snack Cereal & milk Apple	**Snack** Two slices toast Pear or apple	**Snack** Egg sandwich Carton yoghurt, grapes
No Lunch	**No Lunch**	**No Lunch**

Tea
Baked beans on two slices
    toast
Yoghurt
Strawberries
	Tea
	Jacket potato
	Cottage cheese salad
	Banana
		Tea
		Mixed curried vegetables
		    with cubed Bombay
		    Potato
		Stewed apple

Snack Grapes	**Snack** Mango & grapes	**No snack**
Snack One slice bread Sugar-free spread	**Snack** Slice Bran Cake*	**Snack** Banana, strawberries
975 calories	1,121 calories	885 calories

• • • • • • • • •

Suggested 'Snacker's' Menu: Plan Two

Breakfast Cereal Glass fresh orange juice	**Breakfast** Two slices toast Glass fresh orange juice	**Breakfast** Poached egg on two slices toast
Snack Chicken sandwich Apple	**Snack** Apple, peach	**Snack** Handful peanuts Apple
Lunch Two slices crispbread Fruit spread Peach	**Lunch** Mixed salad with vegetable rice	**Lunch** Mixed bean salad Glass fresh orange juice
Snack Carrot & Orange Salad*	**Snack** Banana milk shake	**Snack** Portion semolina pudding
Main Meal Prawn salad	**Main Meal** Fillet steak Broccoli Peas Mushrooms	**Main Meal** Large mixed salad Orange & pawpaw sorbet*
980 calories	985 calories	1,062 calories

Breakfast Slice bread and sugar-free jam	**Breakfast** Glass fresh orange juice	**Breakfast** Cereal One slice toast
Snack Cereal	**Snack** Tuna fish & salad sandwich	**No snack**
Snack One peach One apple	**Snack** Sliced tomatoes Cauliflower Cheese Apple	**Snack** Banana milk shake
Main Meal Beef Goulash Rice Stewed plums	**Main Meal** Chicken Curry with Rice Peach	**Main Meal** Cheese salad Stewed Apple
Snack Orange Slice bread & jam	**Snack** Two crispbreads Banana	**Snack** Pineapple & peach slices
1,032 calories	1,185 calories	897 calories

• • • • • • • • •

Suggested 'Snacker's' Menu: Plan Three

Breakfast ½ grapefruit Home-made muesli with oats, dates, almonds	**Breakfast** ½ grapefruit One slice toast	**Breakfast** Porridge
Snack One slice toast & Marmite	**Snack** Apple, pear	**Snack** Tuna fish sandwich Apple
Snack Cottage cheese with celery & carrot sticks	**Snack** Vegetable soup One slice bread	**Snack** Two-Pear Salad*

Main Meal
Plain cooked penne with
   garlic, olive oil and
   walnuts
Apple
	Main Meal
	Spaghetti with tuna fish &
	   sweetcorn
		Main Meal
		Chicken salad with
		   sweetcorn and colourful
		   vegetables
		Stewed gooseberries &
		   half-fat crème-fraîche

Snack Pear & grapes	**Snack** Grapes	**No snack**
1,263 calories	1,050 calories	1,190 calories

Suggested 'Cheap and Cheerful' Menus

Breakfast Two slices toast Sugar-free jam	**Breakfast** Muesli with oats, almonds and dates	**Breakfast** ½ grapefruit Porridge
Snack Dates & six Brazil nuts	**Snack** Bread & jam Apple	**Snack** Pear
Lunch Cottage cheese & fruit salad Grapes, blueberries Apple	**Lunch** Egg on one slice toast Grapes	**Lunch** Tuna & pasta salad
Snack Bowl porridge	**Snack** Avocado pear with prawns	**Snack** Salad sandwich
Snack Tinned peaches with half- fat crème fraîche	**Snack** Cold chicken salad Pear	**Snack** Apple & grapes
1,055 calories	1,220 calories	1,012 calories

Suggested Wheat-Free Menu Plan

For people who have a mild wheat intolerance.

Breakfast Rice Krispies Glass fresh orange juice	**Breakfast** Corn Flakes Glass fresh orange juice	**Breakfast** Rice Krispies
Lunch Chicken salad Apple	**Lunch** Jacket potato Mixed salad Apple	**Lunch** Spicy Cajun chicken* Peach
Main Meal Chilli Con Carne with Kidney Beans & Rice* Roast pineapple	**Main Meal** Lentil Roast Stewed plums	**Main Meal** Kedgeree* Baked apple with sultanas
Snack Banana	**Snack** Banana, peach	**Snack** Glass fresh orange juice Mixed winter salad
1,340 calories	1,181 calories	1,249 calories
Breakfast Two slices gluten-free toast	**Breakfast** Rice Krispies Glass fresh orange juice	**Breakfast** Corn Flakes Glass fresh orange juice Gluten-free toast
Lunch Chicken & Orange Salad Apple	**Lunch** Lentil & Vegetable Soup Gluten-free bread	**Lunch** Tuna Fish & Rice Salad with Pinto Beans Pineapple & peach salad
Main Meal Braised Beef with Fresh Vegetables Boiled potatoes Rice Pudding	**Main Meal** Grilled salmon Asparagus Puréed carrots Baked Banana*	**Main Meal** Lamb chop Peas Courgettes Carrots
Snack One peach Banana milk shake	**Snack** One apple, one peach	**Snack** Apple
1,361 calories	1,040 calories	1,184 calories

Suggested Menu Plans to Help Chronic Fatigue Sufferers (ME) or Convalescents

ME sufferers have special dietary needs. They tend to gain weight easily and suffer from muscle weakness. On this meal plan, I suggest you choose four main portions of carbohydrate and three pieces of fruit.

Breakfast Cereal Grapefruit segments	**Breakfast** Cereal Prunes	**Breakfast** Cereal Grapefruit
Snack Banana	**Snack** Apple	**Snack** Grapes
Light Lunch Baguette filled with mixed salad Yoghurt & banana, blended	**Light Lunch** Vegetable soup Plain baguette Grapes	**Light Lunch** Teacake Yoghurt with chopped banana & sunflower seeds
Main Meal Roast chicken Jacket potato Carrots & cauliflower	**Main Meal** Spicy Yoghurt-baked Chicken* Naan bread Mixed salad	**Main Meal** Sardines on two slices toasted wholemeal bread
1,369 calories	1,489 calories	1,234 calories

Breakfast Croissant with sugar-free jam	**Breakfast** Cereal Prunes	**Breakfast** Toast Prunes
Lunch Pitta pocket filled with tuna fish & salad Apple	**Lunch** Baguette with prawns & mayonnaise Banana	**Lunch** Wholemeal sandwich with egg & cress Grapes
Main Meal Dry-roasted potatoes, fillet salmon, poached Broccoli, French beans Fresh Fruit Salad*	**Main Meal** Jacket potato Winter Salad*	**Main Meal** Jacket potato with cottage cheese Colourful mixed salad Plain yoghurt
Snack Two slices crispbread Marmite	**Snack** Yoghurt & grapes	**Snack** Cereal with almonds, Brazil nuts & sliced apple
1,440 calories	1,152 calories	1,167 calories

Suggested Arthritis Prevention Menu Plan

This plan does not follow the set patterns of the other menus because there are special considerations. The diet is low in meat and fat, but high in calcium and iron. It also has a high protein of fish, for their essential oils help arthritis sufferers. You may want to try it if you are at risk from arthritis.

Foods to Avoid In Your Diet
- Liver
- Kidneys
- Meat extract
- Red meat
- Tea with meals
- Shrimps
- Anchovies
- Alcohol
- Sugar

Foods To Include In Your Diet
- Lentils (these are rich in iron)
- Cheese
- Semi-skimmed milk
- Low-fat natural yoghurt
- Cottage cheese
- Baked beans
- Boiled cabbage
- White bread
- Salmon

Breakfast Two slices white toast Water or decaffeinated coffee	**Breakfast** Sugar-free muesli Glass fresh orange juice Coffee	**Breakfast** Low-fat natural live plain yoghurt with flaked almonds and chopped apple ½ grapefruit
Lunch Cheese salad to include coloured peppers, carrots & sweetcorn	**Lunch** Mixed salad sandwich Banana	**Lunch** Welsh Rarebit with sliced tomatoes Stewed apple & blackberries with 2 tsp crème fraîche
Main Meal Poached or roast salmon fillet Broccoli, peas or asparagus Three boiled potatoes	**Main Meal** Kedgeree* Mixed fruit salad made from three pieces fruit	**Main Meal** Smoked Salmon on Potato Cakes* & half-fat crème fraîche Caramelized Pear*
Snack Fresh Fruit Salad*	**Snack** Six dried apricots Two slices crispbread	**Snack** Banana
Total calories 1,254	Total calories 1,157	Total calories 1,263

* **Note**: This plan includes a daily allowance of 146 calories for milk and 7g butter.

• • • • • • • • • •

Arthritis Diet

This plan will help those who already suffer from arthritis.

Breakfast Porridge One slice toast with sugar- free jam Coffee	**Breakfast** No-sugar muesli ½ grapefruit Coffee	**Breakfast** Corn Flakes with soya or plain milk *or* two slices toast, sugar-free jam Coffee
Snack Apple	**Snack** Apple	**Snack** Apple, banana
Main Meal Roast chicken Two boiled potatoes Cauliflower, carrots, gravy Rhubarb Sorbet*	**Lunch** Chicken salad Apple	**Lunch** Jacket potato with Smoked Mackerel Fillet & salad
Tea Slice Bran Cake* Fresh Fruit Salad*	**Main Meal** Spaghetti with Smoked Salmon & Dill Sliced peaches & half-fat crème fraîche	**Main Meal** Tuna Fish Salad with French Beans & Sweetcorn Stewed apple, plums or rhubarb
Snack Banana & grapes	**Snack** Banana Shake with soya milk	**Snack** Dairy or soya yoghurt (plain)
Total calories 1,282	Total calories 1,257	Total calories 1,235

The Day of Rest

Everyone needs a break from their diet, a day when you don't have to think about calories, a time to relax in front of the TV, to go to the pub with friends or to simply enjoy a day of catching up with all your chores. You need a break, but you don't need to get fat.

The first week has probably been a bit of 'cold turkey'. Many clients find the first week unbearable because they are still programmed to eating at certain times and in a certain way. Stopping off for a coffee means a slice of cake too, supermarket shopping means a chocolate treat from the range displayed temptingly at the checkout, but these are just simply bad habits which you must break. By the third week you'll have got into the swing of it and found new things to do with your time. You'll also be planning a few cosmetic treats I hope, ready for the newer, slimmer you!

Enjoying yourself doesn't mean eating everything in sight. This has been your problem before and if you are retraining your eating habits you mustn't get out of your routine. Your day off is a day when anything goes, as long as you keep within 2,000 calories. This is the recommended limit to keep an average woman's weight stable without gaining or losing – of course it's over your BMR (basic metabolic rate see pages 44–5) but you are using up calories by simply getting out of bed! You should easily use these up during the course of a day's activities. Today you can have roast potatoes, cakes or biscuits, but don't get carried away. Remember your goal of getting back into those jeans. Think that by the end of this month you'll be much lighter, with a more defined shape you'll be amazed at. A few too many chocolates or crisps at this stage could ruin everything.

Your Calorie Guide (see pages 131–7) has all the answers about calorie values, but try not to get too hung up about it. The most likely way to mount up your calories will be with alcohol, so stick to a limit of three alcoholic drinks per week and no more. It doesn't matter which day out of the seven you choose as your day off. In fact, if you have a special event to go to, count that as your day off – whether it's a Wednesday, Saturday or Monday. But allow yourself just one day – this plan only works if you do it for six days every week.

Keep active. You are reprogramming your body for the future and that means exercise. Go for a walk, run up the stairs, keep busy – a good figure is for life, not just for the New Year!

• • • • • • • • • •

Shaping Back Into Those Jeans

People groan whenever they hear the word 'exercise'. It conjures up images of hard-faced aerobics queens, sweaty games of squash, or tying themselves up in knots at yoga classes. Yet it doesn't have to be like that.

The distribution of your weight is as important to your look as what you weigh. To a certain extent it's down to genetics, but a lot of your shape is also determined by the way you live. Sitting down spreads your bottom and thighs, while manual work can build up shoulders. Hairdressers develop sway backs and protruding stomachs. All of these problems can be helped by regular toning exercise which you should do in your own home as regularly as you would wash your hair.

First Gear – getting going
There are five ways in which you can change your shape:

Everyday Exercise
You get exercise every time you make a movement. Think back to where we discussed your basal metabolic rate (BMR) (see pages 44–5). If you remember, your BMR is based on the calories that your body would use if you were doing nothing. Think of it as a car engine idling, with the speedometer needle set at zero. You put the car into first gear and then begin to move slowly. The needle moves up to five miles an hour and then ten. You change gear, gather speed until you are in top gear at seventy miles an hour and the engine is burning a lot of

• • • • • • • • • •

fuel. Well, your body is like that. From the moment you wake up, your needle is slowly going up. You get out of bed and go downstairs, you make tea and feed the cat. By doing this, you have gathered speed. You have gone from burning one calorie a minute to one and a half. Throughout the day you will be changing gear and either burning more fuel, such as in a brisk run for the train, or slowing down, as you might do by sitting at your office desk. Life may seem hectic in your head, but sitting down at a desk all day burns very few calories. By lunch-time each day, most sedentary workers have consumed far more calories than they have burned off.

Life used to be active because people didn't have the range of labour-saving devices and machines available today. Now we press a switch and flick a button, and our work's done. Compare this with the old days of preparing supper, which would involve washing and peeling vegetables, grating and chopping, and going in and out of the back door to dispose of leftovers. My mother used to be in the kitchen for the whole of Sunday making lunch and tea, but nowadays we put a ready-made meat and two veg. meal into the microwave and it's done in minutes. Salads come in hygienic, no-waste packs, and vegetables are completely prepared for us right down to the cross in the bottom of a sprout. The trouble is: three hours of work was a lot of calories. It's no wonder people get fat when they purchase a dishwasher and give up over two hours of washing-up each week.

I'm not suggesting that we go back to those days – I use a dishwasher too – but if you've outgrown those jeans you need to do something. Just to get you into the swing of things, I have compiled this fun-chart which counts the calories of everyday tasks:

• • • • • • • • • •

Calories Used in a Year

Activity	Calories Used	The Old Way	Calories Used
Changing TV channels with remote control three times in an evening	1,095	Getting up to change channels	2,190
Having someone else make you coffee twice a day, five days a week	1,920	Walking 100 yards to make your own coffee	4,800
Washing your car in a car wash (once a week)	156	Washing your car by hand (thirty minutes)	4,160
Taking your shopping 100 yards to your car in a trolley	600	Carrying heavy shopping to your car twice a week	1,200
Sitting in front of the TV for ten minutes, seven nights a week	3,650	Going for a ten-minute walk seven times a week	18,250
Driving or riding in the bus the whole distance, five days a week, forty-eight weeks a year	240	Parking or alighting five minutes away from your stop and walking the rest of the way (there and back).	12,000
Total:	7,661		42,600

The chart may be for fun, but it is also accurate. These simple tasks add up to a staggering 34,939 *extra* calories used in a year, which is a whole four kilogrammes worth of fat!

Your Goal

You should aim to burn off an extra 150 calories a day through normal activities such as the following:

- fifteen minutes' hand washing
- getting up an hour earlier
- a ten-minute brisk walk to post a letter and back
- eight minutes spent raking leaves or brisk sweeping

Second Gear – Burning Those Calories

Monica's motto

'If it moves, nothing can settle.' Fat loves little corners where it won't be disturbed, so *keep everything moving*! Burning away those calories and fat is what you want to achieve, and you can only do this effectively with aerobic exercise.

Aerobic means 'with air' and it encompasses all the activities that make you slightly breathless and with a faster heartbeat. If you were aiming to be an elite sportsperson I would be talking about percentages of your body's maximum heart rate and volumes of air, but you don't need to worry too much about those sorts of details simply to get back into your jeans! You just want to slice those inches off your thighs and bottom, and one of the most effective ways to deal with fat is through aerobic exercise. The chart that follows below lists all the advantages of aerobic exercise, as well as what it can't achieve.

What Aerobic Exercise *Does*

- Increases heart rate
- Improves circulation
- Burns calories
- Gives you more stamina
- Tones muscles, especially in the lower body.

What it *Doesn't* Do

- Change the shapes of your muscles
- Make your muscles leaner
- Make you more flexible

The best activities for calorie-burning are those which are moderate and long-lasting. Short, hard exercise such as a sprint or racing swimming cannot be endured for hours on end, so although the calories burned are greater per minute than for more moderate exercise, the simple fact that you can go on for longer in exercise such as step aerobics, slow swimming or a day's rambling means that more calories are burned and your system is more efficient.

Turning back to the analogy of a car going through its gears, reaching top gear and settling down into a long motorway run is fuel-efficient and relaxing for the driver. The car works at its best at less than top speed, and so do you. Short, sharp bursts of fast driving cannot be prolonged: they use a lot of fuel and cause wear and tear.

If you're going to get the best from your body you're not going to do it by short, hard games of squash after a day of sitting down. They might exhaust you, but they don't use your fuel efficiently. You need to get into your stride by cycling to work, walking the dog for an afternoon at the weekend or getting on that treadmill and walking briskly for forty-five minutes. Your metabolism stays high for a long time afterwards

• • • • • • • • •

and this matters in weight control and fat burning. In short, sharp bursts you recover quickly, but at the end of longer bouts of moderate exercise your energy supplies are completely out. Eating at this stage is the best way of using your food because it replenishes what you've lost. Unless you eat a really gigantic meal it won't be stored as fat, simply because there won't be anything left as excess.

If you get your exercise in the gym, vary your work-outs between the stairclimber, cycle and treadmill. As you improve and get fitter, don't just make the work-outs longer: make them more intense. Many people can only spare forty-five minutes in the gym at any one time and they cheerfully stick with the same routine, year after year, on auto-pilot. They stagger into gym half asleep, go through their work-out programme, shower and go to work. There is no thought of testing the boundaries, no consideration of variation or intensity. The fact is, if you only have forty-five minutes then that's no problem. As you get fitter and more used to your routine, increase the intensity and not the time spent in the gym. Get the treadmill to climb hills and do the same with the bike, row faster, increase the resistance on the stairclimber. You shouldn't go flat out but you should adjust your work-out. After all, you're fitter now than you used to be!

Here are some basic calorie values:

Basic Calories Used in Exercise

Activity	Calories used per half hour
Walking slowly	120
Walking briskly	180
Walking uphill	240
Playing tennis	210
Jogging	240
Squash	420
Ice skating	150
Aerobics – high impact	195
Aerobics – low impact	165
Gentle cycling	120
Fast cycling	195
Racing cycling	330
Disco dancing	195
Ballroom dancing	105
Golf	165
Horse riding, trotting	210
Netball	210
Slow swimming	255
Fast swimming	300
Medium-paced running	375

Your Goal

The aim is to burn off an *extra* 150 calories a day with an aerobic activity or sport. Here is an example:

Monday	Low-impact aerobics class
Tuesday	Walk to work or have an evening walk
Wednesday	Day off
Thursday	Twenty-minute swim at lunch-time
Friday	Morning or evening walk
Saturday	Game of squash, tennis, football, etc.
Sunday	Cycle ride

Arrange your activities in any way that suits you, but try to get that half hour or so of aerobic exercise on six days of the week. Amazingly, that little bit extra adds up to a staggering 144 *hours*, or six *whole days* of exercise a year, and an even more amazing 43,200 calories, which is 5½ kilogrammes (12 pounds) of your weight gone for good!

What, you don't believe me? Sounds like just a theory? Don't forget that not following this sort of pattern is how your weight crept on in the first place. Take a desk job or give up a manual job for home life and it's a slow decline in activity. Half an hour a day, three hours a week of not being active means that you aren't using up 1,000 calories a week. It all adds up, and suddenly those jeans won't fasten. It's as simple as that.

Third Gear – Toning for a Better Shape

You've burned off fat, but if you're not careful you could end up looking like a rag doll without its stuffing. Fat and muscle are completely different things which simply share a home and, as I said earlier, don't assume your weight is all unwelcome fat. Unless you actually have a fat monitoring machine (and they

• • • • • • • • • •

can be bought in branches of the larger chemists' stores) you won't know how much of your weight is healthy muscle and how much is fat. To give you an idea of how fooled we can be about our fitness, the maximum recommended healthy fat reading for women is 29 per cent. Now, I have a friend, a twig of eight stone (fifty-one kilogrammes) who commends herself on never taking any exercise. But according to my fat monitor she registered a worrying 38 per cent fat! Yes, she was slim, but at the same time unhealthily fat. We have now embarked on a programme to help her lose the fat and replace the weight, whilst filling out her skin with healthy and atttractive-looking muscle.

Toning exercise firms up your muscles, makes them longer and stronger, and gives them definition. It is carried out using your body's own weight – for example, in leg lifts where you are raising your leg against its own weight, which could be as much as 6½ kilogrammes (14 pounds). Toning increases muscle fibres slightly and you will achieve a firmer thigh, a tighter bottom, a flatter stomach and a slimmer waist. Here are the areas you need to work to get back into those jeans:

1 Waist
2 Stomach
3 'Love handles' – the top of the hip bones
4 Inner thighs
5 Outer thighs
6 Front of thighs
7 Backs of thighs
8 Bottom

I shall be dividing your exercises into two groups, which you work on alternate days for balance (see pages 117–19), and to give muscle groups time to recover and improve.

• • • • • • • • • •

Fourth Gear – Sculpting

'Sculpting' is quite a new term. In reality it is simply weight training, but therein lies a problematic image of muscle-bound, hard-faced women with mahogany tans and oiled bodies – fairly off-putting to a lot of us!

But don't be put off. Sculpting is something I do, and I am quite small and not remotely hefty. It means the use of heavier weights for shorter periods of time to increase the size of a particular muscle or to improve its shape and I have followed a programme for two years now to help improve the appearance of my shoulders and arms. Using weights on your legs won't necessarily make them bigger, if you know just how far to go. What they will do is without gaining any extra size, make your legs amazingly tight and hard.

If you really get into a sculpting programme you can say goodbye to any wobble or splay effect. 'Splay' is what happens when you force yourself into too-tight jeans and your spare buttocks splay out to make 'saddlebags'. In your jeans, your bottom will look fantastic!

Someone who went through this plan to test it for me became the envy of her whole office. 'I couldn't believe it,' said a friend, 'there wasn't a bulge anywhere. Her bum was smooth under her jeans with no hint of a droop!' This improvement came about purely through sculpting exercise.

How It Works

Muscle gets bigger by growing more fibres. It does this because it is being forced to work under increasing weights and in resting periods your muscles produce these extra fibres. You can prevent your body from forming huge muscles by limiting the weights you use and stretching your muscles after your work-out.

Don't forget, the more muscle you have the higher your

resting metabolic rate – and the more efficiently you will be burning off calories.

The Warm-up

Always warm up for a few minutes first by walking on the spot or stepping from side to side, swinging your arms, or you could cycle on a stationary bike for five minutes. Stretch out afterwards.

Your Waist – The Forgotten Bit in the Middle

There is one simple exercise for your waist which you do lying on the floor, which you will find on page i of the photo section.

This exercise is effective because it is a stretching movement which tones the oblique muscles. (They run along the side of your torso and shape your waist.)

It's My Stomach!

If you haven't already got my book *5 Days to a Flatter Stomach*, then rush out and buy it now because it has some lovely exercises for you to get your teeth into on this month's plan. It also has specific advice on the other causes of a problem stomach, some of which you may not already have thought of. However, working the stomach can be done with one simple exercise – as long as you promise yourself to do it every day, do all the repetitions and stick with the rules of correct form. You'll find it on page ii of the photo section.

This exercise is so slow that as a guide, you should do no more than four repetitions in a minute.

It's This Bit On My Hips

How many times have I heard that? People come up to me holding bits of flesh with a look of utter despair on their faces, yet that little fleshy 'pad' on the top of your pelvic bones seems to defy all attempts to shift it. And the reason? This area simply doesn't get to move very much in daily life and, as I keep on saying, fat loves little corners where it knows it won't be disturbed.

There is one exercise which I swear by to whittle down that pad and it is, in fact, a stretch. Stick with it. At first you may feel a little stiff the next day and you may also feel that it isn't doing anything – but it is. The stiffness is caused by the muscles in your back and your hips being stretched really thoroughly, probably for the first time. It takes time because these things do. You wouldn't expect your hair to grow back in one week if you'd had it cut too short, and neither will your body change shape miraculously. But by the end of this month, you'll notice a huge difference. Have a look at the instructions on page iii of the picture section.

This exercise is hard to do and you mustn't feel discouraged if you can't go very far. It will come.

Beating Those Saddlebags

I can think of more than a dozen exercises for your outer thighs, but my clients have always told me that nothing worked better than my own invention, an exercise I call 'the curtsey'. It's on page iv of the picture section.

It's not easy, but if you are a complete beginner you can do the simpler version, which is just as effective, and then work up to the full effort. The reason why this movement works so well is because you have to use each leg to raise your whole body weight. I can promise you that when it comes to trimming outer thighs to get back into your jeans, this exercise is the business!

It's best to have some music for this, something which has about 100 beats to the minute. Try and find a suitable piece because it's going to be very useful in the weeks ahead.

• • • • • • • • • •

Inner Thighs

Most of us are unhappy about the shape of our inner thighs. Like hips, they can get out of condition because they are not used very much. The inner thigh muscles are called 'adductors' and they only work when you draw your legs together – not something we do very often! Gripping movements with your thighs, such as in horse riding, are excellent for toning the adductors, but if you are not into riding then you need to make a special effort to tone them.

To get rid of fat on the inner thighs, I recommend the following types of exercise:

- Fast swimming
- Aerobics
- Ballroom dancing
- Ballet
- Tennis
- Football

If you want to shape up flabby, but slim, inner thighs, try the following:

- Floor exercises (see page v of the photo section)
- Horse riding
- Stretching

Fronts of Thighs

If you want to lose weight from large thighs, try the following:

- Fast cycling
- Swimming
- Dancing
- Brisk walking.

• • • • • • • • • •

To shape up untoned slim legs, try the following:

- Floor exercises adding light (450g–1.5kg) ankle weights
- Stretching
- Mountain or resistance cycling
- Step aerobics
- Leg extensions (in the gym)
- Lunges and squats (see below for one version).

Crouching Quadricep Pliés

This is not the most elegant of exercises – but so what? You're in the privacy of your own home and can look as silly as you like. After all, you won't look so silly when the zip on those jeans glides up effortlessly, and all your friends are whispering about your fantastic thighs! The instructions are on page vi of the photo section.

Backs of Thighs

The hamstrings run along the backs of your thighs. Toning them gives an impressive sweep to the backs of your legs and helps to prevent cellulite from developing. The exercise on page vii of the photo section is easy for everyone, although it does take practice. Do as many as you can, going on to the advanced form of the exercise as you get stronger.

The Bottom Line – 'Glute Sweeps'

Your buttock muscles are called 'gluteals' or 'glutes' for short. They are big muscles and they can get out of shape and become slack very quickly. If you stand or sit a lot of the time, you may need firming exercises if you want to have a firm, high bottom.

As with thighs, fast cycling, swimming, skating or hill walking are good fat burners, but toning work to really strengthen and lift the buttocks should be done with resistance. Try any of

the following, or the Glute Sweeps on page viii of the photo
section.

- Hill or mountain cycling
- Step aerobics
- Lunges
- Squats
- Skiing squats
- Standing dips (see page ix of the photo section)

'Glute Bridges'

This exercise can be done by old and young alike, while you're
on the telephone or watching TV. If you like, place a 3–10lb
weight on your hips. It tones and tightens the buttock muscles.
Although it's not photographed, it's very straightforward. Lie
on the floor, knees bent, feet flat on the floor. Being careful not
to arch your back or thrust your pelvis into the air, lift your
buttocks just clear of the floor. Squeeze and release them at a
rate of once a second. Try to do 20 with knees touching, 20
with knees apart, and 20 with heels only on the floor, toes
raised!

Back to Neutral Gear – Stretching Out

Now it's time to cool your engine down and to come back to
where you started. You've burned off a lot of calories and they
will continue to be burned for one to two hours if you've done
vigorous exercise which has lasted over an hour. Stretching
ensures a nice long, lean line to your body and this is essential
if you are to achieve your goal of getting back into those jeans.
Never underestimate the value of stretching. It is as important
to losing weight as diet or aerobics.

• • • • • • • • •

1   Outer Thigh Stretch (see page x of insert)

2   Inner Thigh Stretch (see page x of insert)

3   Quadriceps Stretch (see page x of insert)

4   Hamstring Stretch (see page xi of insert)

5   Gluteal Stretch (see page xi of insert)

6   Waist Stretch (see page xii of insert)

7   Abdominal Stretch (see page xii of insert)

• • • • • • • • • •

Devising a Fitness Programme for your Whole Body

When you start your exercise programme, it's easy to be positive and motivated. By the end of a couple of weeks though, this enthusiasm has often waned. You haven't shrunk two sizes, you haven't lost a stone, you're exhausted and you wonder if it's worth it.

There are two reasons for feeling like this. Going at an exercise programme like a bull at a gate is one thing, and following the same routine day after day is another. However tempted you might be to exercise for two hours a day – don't. Working out a long-term programme means that you won't just stay interested for longer, but you'll reprogramme your body and maintain your fitness level even when resting. Here is an ideal programme to follow:

First Week

Monday
Early morning walk
Aerobics class in the evening or sports session
Floor exercises at home or in the gym:

  Inner Thighs (see page v)
  Outer Thighs ('Curtseys') (see page iv)
  Crouching Pliés (for fronts of thighs) (see page vi)
  Stomach (see page ii)
  Waist Reaches (see page iii)

• • • • • • • • •

Tuesday

Early morning walk *or* thirty minutes on the treadmill at four m.p.h.

Swimming at lunch-time or in the evening

Floorwork:

> Glute Sweeps (see page viii)
> Glute Bridges (see page 115)
> Standing Dips (see page ix)
> Hip Stretch (see page iii)
> Stomach (see page ii)

In the second week, start to use weights to make the exercises a little harder!

Wednesday

This is your day off. Have a walk or easy cycle ride, if possible.

Thursday

Bike ride for forty-five minutes *or* forty-five minutes' brisk or hill walking *or* forty-five minutes on a treadmill at 4.2 m.p.h.

Floorwork, as Monday.

Friday

Thirty minutes early morning walk

Thirty minutes exercise bike (if available) *or* thirty minutes on the stairclimber.

At lunch-time, either walk, swim or go to an exercise class.

Floorwork, as Tuesday.

Saturday

This is your full day off.

• • • • • • • • • •

Sunday

Full programme: Forty-five minutes on an exercise bike *or* a cycle ride. Thirty minutes walking (4.5 m.p.h.) *or* use the stairclimber.

These should all be carried out at moderate pace, with no running or jogging.

Floorwork: A full programme of *all* the exercises, with full sets of repetitions.

Second Week

1   Repeat the programme as for last week allowing a full day off after each two days of exercise.

2   Start to add 450g weights to your ankles for inner thigh exercises, hold weights on hips for Glute Bridges (see page 115).

3   Don't forget to warm up and do a full stretch session after every work-out.

• • • • • • • • •

What Next?

Managing Your Shape for the Future

There is always a feeling that a diet is something which you are either 'on' or 'off'. It achieves the result you want and then it's over. That's no problem if you usually have a stable weight and simply put on a few kilogrammes over Christmas, but if you're a lifelong weight battler you'll need to regard your diet in the same way as you might think of your hairstyle or your dress sense. It's part of your personal style. Your style of eating and the things you eat are your diet and, as far as I know, every smart woman has her own personal diet style. As I told you earlier, I have a diet that works for me. You need to devise a personal diet for the future which takes into account not just the foods you like and dislike, but also the fact that you find food a bit of a temptation!

Having to watch what you eat is no worse than having to watch your hair or having to be careful about your nails. Looking good always has and always will be an effort. People who make no effort, show it. Although I have promised you that no foods are banned, I know you're only human. If you know that once you open that packet of custard creams all hell breaks loose, don't buy them. Life won't stop if you never see the inside of a chip shop again or only savour a prawn vindaloo on your birthday. In any case, it's not that bad. Just keep those foods for special occasions, and you'll appreciate them all the more. You have the willpower, and you have it because you've come this far and the pleasure you'll get from all the compliments about your new figure will far outweigh the fleeting excitement of a bit of cake.

• • • • • • • • • •

Your new regime is more relaxed than the old one because you can choose more carbohydrates. If you want to go back to the menus I devised earlier (see Menus for a Month, pages 68–88) you can choose four from each list and add another protein food. The odd piece of cake won't matter either, because you are still monitoring your calories. This is how you do it.

Calculating Your New Calorie Limits

The good news is that you can now add on a few calories for activity and exercise. This increases your calories from your resting metabolic rate to the normal level, which includes exercise. Activity and exercise will ensure that you don't lose any more weight, but you don't gain it either.

To calculate your new calorie limit, take your old resting rate, e.g. 60 kilogrammes (ten stone) = 1,260 calories a day. Now add on a *third* of this number = 420 calories for moderate activity and your final total will be 1,680. If you are quite active (for example, if you have a manual or walking job) add on a *half* of this number e.g. 1,260 plus 630 = 1,890 calories.

Calculating Your New Carbohydrate Allowance

You can now choose more carbohydrate units. As before, your personal needs depend on several factors: your weight, age, gender and the amount of exercise that you do. Start with your weight in kilogrammes (see page 122 for the calculation) and follow the table according to your general level of activity.

Activity Level	Grammes of Carbohydrate Per kg of Weight
Light (less than an hour a day)	3–4
Moderate (1–2 hours a day)	4–5
Heavy (2–4 hours a day)	5–6

• • • • • • • • •

Note:

Light	Standing or sitting all day, driving, craftwork, light housework, cooking.
Moderate	Walking to and from school or work, shopping, gardening, keep-fit class.
Heavy	Competitive sports, walking for a living (e.g. traffic warden, beat police officer, postman), mountain biking, daily horse riding.

Therefore a 64 kilogrammes (10½ stone) woman doing an office job would need 64 × 3 grammes of carbohydrate a day, which comes to 192 grammes. If she is younger than thirty, she can raise that to 64 × 4 = 256 grammes.

How Do I Know How Much Carbohydrate is in My Food?
Just read the food labels! I have prepared this handy guide to the most common foods that we eat with typical portion sizes. Don't worry, you won't spend the rest of your life weighing and counting. After a while you'll have a good idea of portion sizes even if there isn't a pair of scales in sight.

These Food Portions All Contain 25 grammes of Carbohydrate:

1–2 slices bread	1–2 Weetabix
150g potatoes	40g muesli
75g cooked rice	568ml milk
2 bananas	2–3 apples
150g baked beans	Half slice fruit cake
2–3 oranges	284ml orange juice
2–3 small cartons plain yoghurt	2 bowls (60g) porridge
50g raisins	90g cooked pasta
115g sweetcorn	2 packets crisps
25g chocolate	150g cooked noodles
150g butter beans	140g lentils
4 slices Ryvita	3 tsp honey

So, with an allowance of 192 grammes of carbohydrate, you could make eight choices from this list and add your protein foods.

Sample Menus

Breakfast: Muesli, milk, apple

Lunch: Tuna fish sandwich, banana, packet crisps

Snack: Apple and banana

Main meal: Jacket potato, ham, mixed bean salad, small slice fruit cake, coffee.

Total = 198 grammes of carbohydrate, and 1,498 calories.

Breakfast: Bacon, egg, two slices of bread and butter

Lunch: Coronation Chicken, rice salad, 25g chocolate

Snack: Salad sandwich

Main meal: Lentil and Carrot Soup, Vegetable Lasagne, Fruit Salad.

Total = 197 grammes of carbohydrate and 1,682 calories.

And Finally . . .

I hope you've got back into those old jeans, or that suit or your wedding dress. And I hope you're more confident because of it and will carry on your good work for the future. Look after your new figure. Don't get obsessed about it because it will take care of itself if you remember the golden rules for lasting success:

1   Never ignore hunger. It is your body's way of telling you that it needs food for a reason.

• • • • • • • • • •

2   Never deal with hunger by putting it off with a fizzy drink. Have some starch, such as a slice of bread, instead.

3   Never eat beyond being full. Put your plate aside and finish it in an hour's time – if you still want it.

4   Never go to bed hungry.

5   Never confuse wanting to eat with being hungry. If you have eaten recently then your stomach isn't empty and you are craving food for another reason. Maybe you're bored or lonely? Next time it happens, don't have fruit, try having bread instead.

6   Exercise every day, even if it's just a walk. Think of ways to do extra exercise, such as gardening, going to post a letter or a bit of cleaning – even ten minutes a day adds up.

7   Keep supple with bending and stretching exercises (see pages x–xii).

8   Believe in yourself. No one was born beautiful. If someone looks beautiful it's because he/she looks after themselves. No one has a great body by accident and if you make the same effort you can look great too. It isn't easy but it *is* simple. There's no great mystery to eating less and taking a bit more exercise.

Go for it – and the very best of luck!

'It Was Brilliant!'

As always, I asked a team of volunteers to test out the *Get Back Into Your Jeans Diet* for me. I was fortunate enough to be able to appeal for testers to try it out through my *Sunday Mirror* column and had offers from all over the country. I finally asked 100 people to tell me honestly what they thought.

My aim was not simply to find out if they had lost weight, but also if the diet was practical. After all, I have said that there's a diet out there to suit everybody and in this book I have given you as many options as possible. But at the end of the day, could the volunteers take the food to work, was the whole family able to share meals, and did they find it a chore to keep records?

For the purpose of a more balanced test, twelve of the volunteers were put on a very different type of diet that was also prctical and manageable. But the *Get Back Into Your Jeans Diet* proved far and away the most successful and more important – and the most popular one. Hear what the volunteers had to say:

Eileen, forty-three, is a community midwife in Gloucester

'I was sceptical at first. Being a midwife I am always on the move, and I wasn't sure about being able to keep a diary and look up calories. But I felt unfit and need to lose about 2 stone [12 kilogrammes], so I thought I'd give it a go. The most extraordinary thing for me was discovering how much I'd been eating! I didn't like weighing things at first but I can see now that it's absolutely essential. Thirty grammes of breakfast cereal is less than you think, and I must have been having more than 100 grammes before, thinking it was a normal portion. I didn't like having to restrict my fruit because I eat tons of it usually, but it made me really savour it. In the old days I'd munch an apple while driving and not even remember eating it.

'This diet made me aware of what I was eating and now I don't have to write down anything at all. In one month I went down from a size 16 to a 14, and now I've lost another 6 pounds [2¾ kilogrammes] in the second month. My aim was to get back into a favourite holiday dress, and I can! I'm absolutely thrilled.'

• • • • • • • • • •

Jenni, twenty-three, is a research scientist in Cambridge

'It was brilliant. I'd gained weight very quickly since getting this job a year ago, I think because of all the standing around I do now, whereas before I was quite active. I hadn't appreciated how the lack of exercise mounted up with time, especially as I don't really eat a lot. I suppose I thought I was slim for life.

'I really took the exercise message on board, and tried to increase it by starting to walk to work. I decided to stop having my newspaper delivered and now walk to the shop for it each morning. The diet was terrific because it made me decide what to eat for a week in advance, so I went to the shops with a proper list and didn't deviate from it, or eat unnecessarily 'on the hoof'. I knew I should be doing that anyway, but you don't always think about it, do you? I used to go home and then wonder what to eat and the cupboard would be bare so I'd pop out for a takeaway. Now I have a lot of home-made food ready-prepared in the fridge. I've lost a stone [6 kilogrammes] in one month, and I'll never go back to the way I was before. I feel so good.'

Elsa, sixty-two, is a retired supervisor from County Down:

'I have very bad arthritis, so I can't exercise. I'm housebound so meals mean a lot to me. What I liked about this diet was that there was a special diet for arthritis sufferers which helped a lot. I'd been given all sorts of leaflets but they don't really tell you in detail how to plan your meals. I found myself feeling a lot less stiff and able to walk a bit each morning, which I hadn't done for ages. A lot of diets suggest ready-made meals, but not everyone wants fast food. It was like putting together a jigsaw, deciding what to eat with what, but as I have time I enjoyed it.

'One big bonus was that I slept a lot better. I used to feel guilty about eating a sandwich late, but I had one every night on the diet and still lost weight. I've been able to get back into a really favourite skirt, and although I only lost 5 pounds [2¼ kilogrammes], my clothes are really loose and that's what makes me feel so ecstatic.'

Helene is thirty-two and a housewife in Cardiff

'I get pretty frazzled having five children under the age of ten. To be honest, I think that trying to cope with having a coherent plan for looking after myself is why I was so fat. I ate all the time. I found it really hard to stick with the *Get Back Into Your Jeans Diet* at first, simply because I am used to putting bits of food into my mouth all the time. I nearly gave up. After a week, though, I understood what Monica meant about retraining yourself. My first reactions were really just withdrawal symptoms. As soon as I realized all that eating was just a habit, and that my weight was going down, I felt much more positive. I lost 12 pounds [5½ kilogrammes] in the month and increased my exercise a lot. I've got back into my jeans which I didn't think I ever would again. They didn't fit on my thighs before, but now they're loose. I can't tell you how good it feels to be a mum-of-five getting back into the jeans I wore before I had the children!'

Janis, forty, is a personal finance adviser from York:

'What I am most pleased about is the way my body has toned up. I didn't think a few exercises at home would make any difference, but even my husband has commented on my firmer bottom and slimmer stomach. I'm over the moon! I didn't necessarily want to lose much weight, but I knew I was eating rubbish and felt tired all the time, and had a feeling a sensible diet like this would be a real bonus. I feel great and ready for anything – so full of life. I'd recommend this diet and exercise plan to anyone.'

• • • • • • • • • •

Anita, twenty-four, is a marketing manager from Jersey:

'This was the best diet I've ever been on. It was brilliant! Although I had to think about it, I also felt that the hassle had been taken out of it by the carbohydrates being counted and the portions laid out. I admit that I have a lot of weight to lose as I'm over 17 stone [102 kilogrammes] and want to be a size 12, but this plan gave me so much encouragement. I always thought it would be impossible for me to aim so high, but now I know I can. I used to wonder why I kept a favourite suit in the wardrobe – it's gone everywhere with me for years now – but now I know I'll get back into it. I've lost 16 pounds [7 kilogrammes] and I'm thrilled.'

Tania, thirty-five, has her own jewellery business in London:

'I really am the last of the terrible eaters. I sit all day designing jewellery and have a coke and a bun on the go all the time. I get tired a lot and I work long hours, so I'm sometimes still picking after midnight.

'This diet made me want to go for it. I know it isn't the diet which does the work, it's you, but that has always been my downfall – lack of willpower. For the first time in my life I have stuck at something for six weeks and I feel it's part of my life now. I liked the way I could choose my own meals or follow the suggestions, and I did both. Being a picky eater and a lousy cook, I stuck with the diet which has a lot of bread in it, and I was amazed at how much bread I ate and still lost weight!

'I also go home now and have a walk without fail. I take a lunch break and have a walk then too. I never eat absent-mindedly. I make a time to stop, and I stop, even if it's only for fifteen minutes. I never knew about sugar and the amounts in the food you buy, and I've become a bit of a Sherlock Holmes on the quiet now – checking labels and boring everyone with my knowledge! My tiredness has completely vanished and I'm

• • • • • • • • •

working a lot more efficiently. This has been the big breakthrough.

'I lost 11 pounds [5 kilogrammes], and the best part has been getting back into some particularly sexy black trousers which I love. It's really cheered me up.'

Lucy is nineteen and a hairdresser from Cheltenham:

'I've lost over a stone [6 kilogrammes] for my wedding. What I can't believe is that I've stopped thinking I need to weigh myself five times a day, which I never thought possible. I simply don't care about what I weigh any more, because I look slim and I feel slim, and that's all that matters. I have learned to understand calories and Monica is right – after a couple of weeks I didn't need to look anything up because I'd come to know the calories in what I myself ate. I'm not fixated, and I'll have a cake if I want one now. The only thing is that now, I *don't* want one!

'I was really keen to get back into my favourite jeans for my new life as a married woman. They're a really great fit and I couldn't believe it when the zip went up easily. It was all in my bottom, and I've lost it!'

• • • • • • • • •

Your Calorie Guide

Calorie Values of your Basic Foods

Use this table as a ready-reckoner for the values of your basic foods. It will help you as you compile your own menus, and explain the calorific content of the ones I've suggested.

Item	Calories per 28 grammes
Bread	
1 medium slice granary	80
1 medium slice wholemeal	75
1 thick slice granary	95
1 thick slice wholemeal	90
(all per 28g slice)	
Malt loaf	76
Ciabatta	73
Olive or tomato bread	80
Foccacia	82
Rye Bread	62
Baguette (100g)	210
Ryvita multigrain, slice	28
Croissant (each)	230
Teacake (each)	230
Naan bread, whole	370
Pitta bread, one	170

Cakes

Fruit scone, average	160
Flapjack	200
Slice sponge cake	120
Rich fruit cake (100g)	280
Meringue nest	65

Cereals (per 30g serving)

Bran Flakes or Sultana Bran	90
Sugar-free muesli	101
Porridge oats	107
Shredded Wheat, each	75
Rice Krispies	105
Weetabix, each	65
Grape nuts	95
Ready Brek	102
Special K	105

Dairy Produce (per 28g)

Butter	224
Eggs, each	85
Cheddar cheese	120
Edam	94
Cheshire	110
Cottage	33
Crème fraîche (half fat), per dsp	52
Whole milk, per 568ml	380
Semi-skimmed	260
Skimmed	190
Bio yoghurt, plain, 150ml	88

Fish (per 28g)

Haddock, hake, cod	25
Mackerel, grilled	68
Mackeral (tinned) in tomato	58
Mackerel (tinned) in oil	70
Prawns	28
Fresh or frozen salmon	55
Smoked salmon	40
Sardines in oil, drained	62
Sardines in tomato	46
Tuna in oil, drained	54
Tuna in brine or water	28

Fruit

Apples, each	55
Avocado pear, half	130
Banana, each	90
Blackberries or blackcurrants, per 28g	8
Cherries, fresh, per 28g	11
Damsons or plums	8
Grapefruit, per half	30
Grapes, seedless	17
Grapes, each	3
Mango, fresh	16
Mango, per whole fruit	105
Melon, half fruit	55
Orange, medium	45
Peach	45
Pear	45
Rhubarb, stewed, no sugar	2
Raspberries	7
Strawberries	8

Fruit, Dried

Apricots, each	10
Currants (per 28g)	76
Dates, each	15
Figs	45
Prunes, each	10

Meat and Poultry (per 28g)

Beef	35
Chicken (leg or breast), roasted	42
Ham (lean) boiled	47
Lamb (lean) roasted	58
Lamb chop	200
Mince, extra-lean	50
Pork (lean) roasted	52
Pork chop, average	170
Steak, fillet or sirloin	50

Nuts (per nut)

Almonds	10
Brazils	20
Hazelnuts	10
Walnuts	40

Vegetables (per 28g)

Aubergines	4
Asparagus, spear	5
Broccoli	7
Cabbage	5
Carrots	7
Cauliflower	8
Leeks	6
Peas	19

Sprouts	10
Parsnips	19
Potatoes	25
Spinach	5
Broad beans	14
Butter beans	29
Green beans	8
Kidney beans	27
Baked beans	23

Extras
1 tsp sugar	10
1 tsp golden syrup	30

Pasta (per 28g)
Fresh, all shapes	80
Dry, all shapes	98
Boiled, all shapes	32

Rice
Brown or white, raw	105
Boiled	40
Semolina or tapioca, raw	100

Salads
Beetroot	13
Cucumber	3
Courgette	5
Carrot	10
Salad greens	4
Onions	10
Radishes	2
Sweetcorn	25

• • • • • • • • •

Tomatoes, each	15
Watercress	6
1 tsp mayonnaise	40
1 tbsp French dressing	80
1 tbsp tomato paste	10
1 tbsp tomato ketchup	15
1 tbsp Ploughman's pickle	20
1 tbsp salad cream	35
1 tbsp Thousand Island dressing	65
1 tbsp prawn cocktail dressing	65

Eating Out
Indian

Chicken Tikka with a half portion of boiled rice	495
Tandoori chicken with a half portion of rice	450
Mixed Vegetable Curry with a half portion of rice	605
Poppadums, each	65

Chinese

Chicken and Sweetcorn Soup	170
Crab and Sweetcorn Soup	150
Prawn Crackers, each	15
Sesame Prawn Toasts, each	70
Beef in Oyster Sauce with a half portion of boiled rice	500
King Prawns with tomatoes, bean sprouts & a half portion of rice	560
Prawn Chop Suey with a half portion of rice	465

McDonald's

Hamburger with Regular fries	510
Filet O' Fish with Regular fries	615
Six Chicken McNuggets, Barbecue sauce	315

• • • • • • • • •

Strawberry Trifle	185
Regular Milkshake	365

Pizza Hut
(deep pan, eighth of a medium pizza)

Cheese	246
Pepperoni	270
Supreme	295
Super Supreme	282

(Personal pan pizza)

Pepperoni	338
Supreme	324

(Thin 'n' crispy slice)

Cheese	199
Pepperoni	207
Supreme	230
Super Supreme	232

Steak Bars & Carveries

Melon	60
Tomato Soup	150
Chicken Satay	190
Fillet steak, Jacket Potato, Sour Cream & Vegetables	535
Fillet Steak, French Fries & Vegetables	685
Garlic Chicken, Fries & Peas	705
Vegetable Bake (Harvester)	605
Salmon Mesquite, Jacket Potato & Peas	670
Pasta & Vegetable Bake	350
Deep-fried Plaice with Tartare Sauce, Jacket Potato & Salad	760

• • • • • • • • •

Recipes for Success

Here are all the recipes for the menus I've suggested on pages 140–78. Combine them with your own favourite dishes – as long as you've made sure they are within your calorie limits – or following whole plans through.

Recipes
The recipes planned in this chapter are all organized alphabetically as follows:

• • • • • • • • • •

• • • • • • • • •

Baby Balti Vegetables

Serves 2   Calories per Serving 132

Ingredients

8 small new potatoes

8 baby carrots

2 tbsp vegetable or corn oil

8 very small onions

1 tsp ginger paste

1 tsp garlic purée or 1 crushed garlic
  clove

1 tsp chilli sauce

1 small tin (125g) chickpeas

8 small courgettes or 2 standard
  courgettes, sliced

8 mangetouts

8 baby sweetcorn

8 cherry tomatoes

1 tsp dried and crushed chillies

2 tsp sesame seeds

Naan bread, to serve

Method

1 Bring a pan of water to the boil and add the potatoes and carrots. Boil for 5 minutes and drain.

2 Heat the oil in a large frying-pan or wok over a high heat. Add the onions and fry until golden brown.

3 Lower the heat and add the ginger paste, garlic purée or crushed garlic and chilli sauce.

4 Add the chickpeas and stir-fry for 2 minutes until all the moisture has been absorbed.

5 Next, add the cooked potatoes and carrots, plus the courgettes, mangetouts, baby sweetcorn and tomatoes. Stir constantly over the heat for a further 2 minutes.

6 Finally, add the crushed chillies, turn onto a serving plate and sprinkle with the sesame seeds. Serve with Naan bread.

• • • • • • • • •

Baked Banana

Serves 2   Calories per Serving 140 (with Crème Fraîche 199)

Ingredients

2 bananas, skinned

Juice from 2 oranges

1 measure Grand Marnier or Cointreau
   (optional)

2 tbsp half-fat fromage frais

Method

1 Preheat the oven to 200°C/400°F/Gas Mark 6.

2 Lay the bananas in a shallow, ovenproof dish. Pour over the orange juice and liqueur, if using.

3 Bake in the centre of the oven, uncovered, for 10–15 minutes.

4 Serve with fromage frais.

Baked Brie Ciabatta

Serves 4   Calories per Serving 407

Use goat's cheese or a garlic and herb cream cheese as an alternative to the Brie.

Ingredients

3 large tomatoes, sliced

Seasoning, to taste

1 garlic clove, halved

2 ciabatta loaves, halved lengthways

175g young spinach leaves

½ tbsp olive oil

225g Brie, thinly sliced

Method

1 Preheat the grill to hot. Put the tomatoes onto a baking sheet and season with salt and freshly ground black pepper. Cook for 5 minutes until softened and hot.

2 Meanwhile, rub the cut edge of the garlic clove over the cut surface of the ciabatta, then cut each piece of the ciabatta into three portions.

3 Preheat the oven to 220°C/425°F/Gas 7. Toss the spinach leaves in the olive oil and use the mixture to cover eight of the ciabatta pieces.

4 Top with the Brie and tomatoes. Place the topped ciabatta in piles of two, then top with the remaining plain ciabatta to make four triple-deck sandwiches.

5 Place the sandwiches on a large baking sheet and bake for 6–8 minutes until the cheese has melted slightly. Serve immediately.

Beef Goulash

Serves 4   Calories per Serving 342

Ingredients

1 tbsp oil	1 × 450g tin chopped tomatoes
450g best braising steak, cubed	225g mushrooms, sliced
1 onion, chopped	1 red pepper, sliced into rounds
1 clove garlic, crushed (optional)	1 tbsp paprika
1 tbsp cornflour	2 tbsp half-fat crème fraîche
300ml red wine	Seasoning, to taste
150ml plain water	Green vegetables and rice, to serve

Method

1 Preheat the oven to 170°C/325°F/Gas Mark 3.

2 Put the oil into a large frying-pan over a low heat and heat until moderately hot, add the beef and turn quickly for about 2 minutes to 'seal' it, until brown on all sides.

3 Add the onion and garlic, and continue to fry gently until the onion is transparent.

4 Turn down the heat, add the cornflour and toss until the meat and onions are thoroughly coated.

5 Transfer to a large ovenproof casserole dish and add the red wine and water. Cover and place in the oven. Cook for 1 hour.

6 Remove from the oven and add the tinned tomatoes, mushrooms and red pepper. Cook for a further 1½ hours.

7 Test the meat by removing one cube and cutting into it. It should fall apart quite easily. If it is not ready, return to the oven for a further 30 minutes.

8 When ready, allow to cool slightly for 5 minutes, then add the paprika and stir in the crème fraîche. Season as necessary, and serve immediately with green vegetables and rice.

Bombay Potato Salad

Serves 2   Calories per Serving 148

Ingredients

450g small new potatoes, scrubbed	Seasoning, to taste
½ tsp ground coriander	1 green chilli pepper, de-seeded and
½ tsp ground cumin	chopped (optional)
75ml Greek yoghurt	Sprigs of parsley, chopped, to garnish

Method

1 Cook the potatoes in boiling, salted water for 15–20 minutes until tender.

2 To make the dressing, whisk together the spices, yoghurt, salt and pepper.

3 Drain the potatoes, leave to cool very slightly and stir into the dressing. Leave to cool completely, then cover and refrigerate until 20 minutes before required.

4 Before serving, stir in the chilli. Garnish with parsley.

Bran Cake

Makes 10 slices   Calories per Slice 188

This cake is fat-free, sugar-free and egg-free. The sweetness comes from the heavy concentration of dried fruits and it has a wonderfully nutty flavour and texture from the walnuts, almonds and seeds

---

Ingredients

50g All Bran

300ml skimmed milk

200g sultanas

Butter or margarine, for greasing

100g dried apricots, halved

2 tbsp sugar-free marmalade

100g walnuts

50g flaked almonds

50g sesame seeds

50g sunflower seeds

100g white self-raising flour, sifted

Method

1 Put the All Bran into a large mixing bowl and cover with the milk.

2 Add the sultanas and dried apricots and stir. Leave to soak for at least one hour.

3 Heat the oven to 180°C/350°F/Gas Mark 4 and grease and line a 450-g loaf tin.

4 When the All Bran mixture has been thoroughly soaked and softened, add the marmalade and combine well. Add the nuts, sesame seeds, sunflower seeds and flour. Stir well and turn into the loaf tin. Bake in the centre of the preheated oven for about 45 minutes or until a skewer inserted into the middle of the loaf comes out clean. If the loaf is not ready, return to oven for a further 15 minutes.

5 When cooked, allow to cool in the tin. Wrap in foil and store in a tin in a cool place. Keeps for about a week.

Cannelloni Stuffed with Spinach & Almonds

Serves 4   Calories per Serving 474

Ingredients

Olive oil

12–16 sheets fresh cannelloni

900g frozen spinach, thawed

100g ground almonds

6 tbsp half-fat crème fraîche

Seasoning, to taste

55g grated Gruyère or Mozzarella
   cheese

Butter, for greasing

55g grated Parmesan cheese

Mixed green salad, to serve

Method

1 Preheat the oven to 150°C/300°F/Gas Mark 2.

2 In a large pan of boiling water with 2 teaspoons olive oil, cook the cannelloni following the instructions on the package. When cooked, drain and serve.

3 Squeeze out any excess water from the spinach and place it in a bowl. Add the almonds, 2 tablespoons of the crème fraîche, seasoning and the Gruyère or Mozzarella cheese. Mix well to combine.

4 Take one sheet of the cannelloni and lay a portion of the spinach mixture on top of it. Roll it up, tucking in the ends. Do the same for the remainder of the cannelloni and stuffing.

5 Butter an ovenproof dish. Place the cannelloni inside it, side by side, to fit snugly. Cover with the remaining 4 tablespoons crème fraîche. Sprinkle with the Parmesan cheese and bake in the middle of the oven for about 20 minutes. Serve piping hot with a mixed green salad.

Caramelized Pear

Serves 2   Calories per Serving 155

Ingredients

1 tsp butter

2 pears, peeled, cored and cut in half

2 tsp sugar

1 tsp five-spice powder

Low-fat fromage frais, to serve

Method

1 Melt the butter in a non-stick frying pan. Add the pears, sugar and five-spice powder.

2 Heat through gently, stirring occasionally. When the fruit is tender and slightly caramelized, remove it with a slotted spoon and serve it on warmed serving plates with 1 tablespoonful of fromage frais per person.

Carrot and Orange Salad

Serves 2   Calories per serving 62

Ingredients

2 large oranges

2 medium carrots

Bunch watercress, washed

2 dessertspoons standard French dressing

30g pine kernels or sunflower seeds, toasted

Method

1 Peel the oranges with a knife so that no pith is left. Slice horizontally into very thin slices.

2 Peel the carrots. Using a potato peeler, peel long thin 'ribbons' down the side of each carrot. It might take a few tries to perfect the procedure, alternatively you could use the slicing side of a standard grater.

• • • • • • • • • •

3 Arrange bunches of watercress on plates, toss the combined orange slices and carrot ribbons in the French dressing and pile onto the watercress. Just before serving, sprinkle a small handful of toasted seeds on top of each salad.

This salad is delicious served with plain grilled chicken, poached white fish or plain crusty French bread.

Chilli Con Carne

Serves 4   Calories per Serving 233

Ingredients

450g extra-lean mince	1 × 450g tin kidney beans
1½ tbsp vegetable oil	1 green chilli, de-seeded and cut into
1 small onion, finely chopped	thin rounds
1 clove garlic, crushed	1 tsp hot or mild chilli powder, to taste
1 × 250g tin tomatoes, chopped with	Seasoning, to taste
herbs	Plain boiled rice and green salad or
2 tbsp concentrated tomato paste	vegetables, to serve

Method

1 In a large frying pan, fry the mince without any added fat or oil until the fat runs clear. Drain and set the meat aside.
2 Heat the oil and gently sauté the onion until softened. Drain away any excess oil. Add the mince, garlic, tomatoes and tomato paste. Turn down the heat, cover the pan and simmer for 5 minutes.
3 Next, add the chilli, kidney beans and chilli powder, if liked, to the mince mixture. Stir and continue to simmer for a further 10 minutes.
4 Check the seasoning and add salt and pepper, if necessary. Serve with a portion of plain boiled rice and a green salad or vegetables.

• • • • • • • • • •

Courgette & Tomato Gratin

Serves 2   Calories per Serving 308

Ingredients

28g butter

2 tbsp vegetable oil

675g courgettes, thinly sliced

1 medium onion, chopped

1 clove garlic, crushed (optional)

450g chopped, tinned tomatoes

Seasoning, to taste

50g soft fresh breadcrumbs, mixed
    with a handful of dried herbs

28g Cheddar cheese, grated

Jacket potatoes or grilled chicken, to
    serve

Method

1 Preheat the oven to 200°C/400°F/Gas Mark 6.

2 Melt half the butter with 1 tablespoonful of the oil in a large saucepan over medium heat, add the courgettes, cover and cook for 5 minutes.

3 Heat the remaining oil in another medium-sized pan, add the onion, cover and cook for 5 minutes, stirring occasionally. Add the garlic and cook for a further 2 minutes.

4 Reduce the heat under the pan containing the onions, add the tomatoes, cover and cook for 5 minutes. Season well with salt and pepper.

5 Stir the courgettes into the tomato mixture and pour into a shallow, well-greased ovenproof dish. Level the top, sprinkle with the breadcrumbs and cheese, and dot with the remaining butter.

6 Bake, uncovered, for about 25–30 minutes until the top is golden brown and crisp. Serve with jacket potatoes or grilled chicken.

• • • • • • • • •

Feta & Walnut Salad

Serves 4   Calories per Serving 393

This simple hot salad makes a light supper.

Ingredients

350g baby new potatoes or cubed old
  potatoes
2 tbsp vegetable oil
115g baby corn, halved lengthways
100g tinned broad beans
Salad leaves

50g walnuts, chopped
Grated peel of one orange
350g feta cheese, cubed
3 tbsp parsley, roughly chopped
Warm walnut bread, to serve

Method

1 Boil the potatoes for about 10 minutes or until done. Drain and reserve. If using the whole new potatoes, slice into rounds.

2 In a large frying-pan, heat the oil. Add the baby corn, broad beans and potato slices or cubes. Stir-fry the vegetables and beans in the oil over a medium heat for 3 minutes, browning the potatoes.

3 Line a dinner plate with a bed of salad leaves.

4 Add the chopped walnuts to the mixture in the frying pan and heat through. Then add the grated orange peel.

5 Remove the pan from the heat, quickly add the feta cheese cubes and combine. Turn onto the salad leaves, garnish with chopped parsley and serve immediately with warm walnut bread.

Fresh Fruit Salad

Serves 4   Calories per Serving 133 (with crème fraîche, 183)

Ingredients

2 bananas	100g fresh pineapple segments
2 apples, washed	100g blueberries, washed
juice of one lemon	other fresh fruit in season, eg
1 grapefruit	strawberries, raspberries
40 seedless grapes, washed	juice of two oranges

Method

1 Peel and slice the bananas. Core and slice the apples, leaving the skins on. Place in a bowl with the lemon juice, and turn to coat well.

2 Halve the grapefruit and using a grapefruit knife, remove the half-segments cleanly. Discard any pips, but take care to keep all the juice. Add to the bananas and apples.

3 Halve the grapes (leave the skins on) and add, along with the pineapple segments, blueberries and any other fruits.

4 Pour over the juice of the two oranges. Mix well and refrigerate before serving. Serve with a tablespoon half fat crème fraîche (optional).

• • • • • • • • • •

Home-made Fresh Vegetable Soup

Serves 4   Calories per Serving 90

Ingredients

225g ripe tomatoes

1 tbsp vegetable oil

1 medium onion, finely chopped

2 medium carrots, chopped

4–6 cauliflower florets

Handful french or runner beans, stringed

2 large potatoes, peeled and cut into small dice

1 bay leaf

½ tsp ground coriander

450ml vegetable stock

Salt and freshly ground black pepper

50ml low-fat crème fraîche

Method

1 Cut a cross in each tomato and immerse in boiling water for 30 seconds. Dip briefly into cold water, then remove and slip off the skins. Chop into quarters.

2 Heat the oil in a non-stick frying-pan and add the onion. Stir over a medium heat until soft. Transfer the onion to a saucepan and add the carrots, cauliflower, beans, potatoes and tomatoes. Add the bay leaf, coriander, stock, a little salt and plenty of black pepper. Cover and simmer for 20 minutes.

3 Allow the soup to cool a little, then remove the bay leaf and transfer the soup to a blender. If desired, reserve a few vegetables to serve as pieces in the soup. Adjust the seasoning and reheat, swirling the crème fraîche into the soup just before serving.

Hot Spiced Oranges

Serves 2   Calories per Serving 165

Ingredients

2 large oranges, peeled and cut into
   segments
1 tsp butter
1 measure Cointreau
Juice and zest of two more oranges

6 cloves
½ tsp cinnamon
2 tsp sugar
Fromage frais, to decorate

Method

1 Preheat the oven to 200°C/400°F/Gas Mark 6.

2 In a buttered, shallow ovenproof dish, place the orange segments and pour the Cointreau and orange juice over the top. Stir in half of the orange zest, and add the cloves and cinnamon. Sprinkle with sugar.

3 Cover the dish with foil and bake in the oven for 15–20 minutes.

4 Remove the dish from the oven, transfer to pudding bowls and decorate with a sprinkling of orange zest and fromage frais.

Kedgeree

Serves 2   Calories per Serving 390

Ingredients

450g smoked haddock fillets

150ml skimmed milk, for poaching

100g Basmati rice

8g butter

½ onion, finely chopped

1–2 teaspoons curry powder

1 tsp ground turmeric

2 hard-boiled eggs, chopped

Seasoning, to taste

A handful of fresh parsley, chopped, to garnish

Crusty French bread or watercress salad, to serve

Method

1 Place the haddock in a large frying-pan and cover with milk. Poach gently for 10 minutes until cooked through. Remove the fish and set aside. Reserve the milk in the pan.

2 Meanwhile, set the rice to boil according to the instructions on the packet. When ready, drain and reserve.

3 In another frying-pan, gently sauté the onion in the butter. Add the cooked rice, curry powder and turmeric, and stir well until incorporated. Pour the reserved milk into the mixture and heat gently.

4 Flake the cooked haddock into large pieces and add to the rice mixture. Add the hard-boiled eggs and turn onto a warm serving dish.

5 Garnish with parsley, adjust the seasoning and serve hot, with crusty French bread or a watercress salad.

Lasagne Verdi

Serves 4   Calories per Serving 354

Ingredients

1 tbsp oil	1 carton half-fat crème fraîche
10–12 sheets lasagne	225g Sage Derby cheese, grated
680g leaf spinach	30g fresh white breadcrumbs
28g butter	115g fresh Parmesan cheese, grated
Seasoning, to taste	30g parsley, chopped
Butter, for greasing	Green salad, to serve

Method

1 Fill a saucepan half full of boiling water and 1 tablespoonful of oil, and cook the lasagne until soft. Drain.

2 Remove the stalks from the spinach and cook in the butter for about 5 minutes until soft. Remove from the heat and season with salt and pepper.

3 Pre-heat the oven to 190°C/375°F/Gas Mark 5.

4 Butter a large ovenproof dish and line the bottom and sides with half the lasagne. Cover with half the spinach mixture, half the crème fraîche and a final layer of lasagne.

5 Next, cover the final layer of lasagne with the remaining crème fraîche, Sage Derby cheese, breadcrumbs and Parmesan cheese.

6 Bake in the oven for 40 minutes. Garnish with parsley and serve immediately with a green salad.

Lentil Roast

Serves 2   Calories per serving 460

Ingredients

225g red or brown lentils, washed
   (soak brown lentils overnight)
60g butter
1 large onion, chopped
3 tomatoes, chopped

60g cornflakes, crushed
115g Cheddar cheese, grated
Salt and pepper
Mixed herbs, parsley and celery salt,
   to taste

Method

1 Heat oven to 180°C/350°F/Gas Mark 4. Grease a 1½ pint loaf tin.

2 Drain the lentils. Put them in a saucepan with ½ pint/285 ml water and bring to the boil. Cover the pan and reduce heat. Simmer until the lentils are soft and the water is absorbed.

3 In a frying-pan, fry the onion in the butter until soft but not brown. Add the tomatoes and cook for 5 minutes. Mash the lentils, add the cornflakes, the onion mixture and the remaining ingredients. Adjust the seasoning.

4 Turn into the loaf tin and sprinkle with a little more grated cheese. Bake for 30 minutes. Serve with a mixed salad or fresh steamed vegetables.

Lentil & Tofu Stir-Fry

Serves 2   Calories per Serving 475

Ingredients

3 tbsp soy sauce

3 tbsp sherry

1 garlic clove, crushed

Small piece root ginger, grated

250g tofu, cubed

4 tsp sesame oil

2 courgettes, cut into matchsticks

100g mushrooms, sliced

1 × 400g tin green lentils, drained

Seasoning, to taste

Boiled rice, to serve

Method

1 Mix together the soy sauce, sherry, garlic and ginger in a bowl. Add the tofu and stir until coated. Leave to marinate for about 10 minutes.

2 Heat half the sesame oil in a large frying-pan. Drain the tofu, reserving the marinade, and fry for 5 minutes until golden. Remove and keep hot.

3 Heat the remaining oil, add the vegetables and stir-fry. Add the lentils, tofu and reserved marinade, and cook for a further 3 minutes. Season and serve with boiled rice.

• • • • • • • • •

Mango or Orange or Raspberry & Rhubarb Sorbet

Serves 4   Calories per Serving 110

Ingredients

4 mangoes or 4 oranges or 225g   4 egg whites
  raspberries or 225g rhubarb   56g caster sugar

Method

1 For Mango Sorbet, peel the mangoes and slice the flesh away from the core. Mash in a bowl or liquidize for 30 seconds until pulped.

If you are making Orange Sorbet, remove the zest from the oranges and extract the juice. Mix both together in a medium-sized bowl.

For Raspberry & Rhubarb Sorbet, peel the rhubarb and remove the stalks from raspberries. Chop the rhubarb and put it into a pan with the raspberries and 1 tablespoonful water to prevent burning. Simmer until the fruit is very soft, about 5 minutes. Leave to cool.

2 In a medium bowl, whisk the egg whites until stiff but not dry. Gradually add the sugar, one tablespoonful at a time, whisking between each spoonful. When all the sugar is added, continue whisking until the meringue forms stiff peaks.

3 Fold the meringue into your chosen fruit, being careful not to beat it. Slowly incorporate the two. Turn into a freezer container and freeze immediately.

4 Remove after 1 hour and stir the sorbet. Freeze for a further 2 hours and stir again. Remove from freezer 20 minutes before serving to soften slightly.

• • • • • • • • •

Pasta Twists with Pesto and Nut Dressing

Serves 4   Calories per Serving 325

Ingredients

200g fresh pasta twists, ideally
  multicoloured (white, red and green)
  (you can buy multicoloured pasta
  twists in the dried pasta ranges)
500ml olive oil
100ml wine vinegar

1 tsp caster sugar
Salt and freshly ground black pepper
1 tsp Dijon mustard
2 tbsp green pesto sauce
100g pine nut kernels, toasted
Large handful rocket leaves

Method

1 Cook the pasta according to the directions on the packet.

2 Meanwhile, prepare the dressing. In a bowl, combine the olive oil, vinegar, sugar, salt and pepper (to taste), mustard and pesto. Whisk together for a minute. Add the pine nuts and the rocket.

3 Turn the hot pasta into a very hot serving dish, add the sauce and combine quickly. Serve immediately on its own, or with plain chicken which has been cut into thin strips and stir-fried.

Alternatively, you can serve with toasted hazelnuts, walnuts or almond flakes.

Pear & Apple Charlotte

Serves 4   Calories per Serving

Ingredients

1 tbsp water

350g baking apples, peeled and cut
 into chunks

350g pears, peeled and cut into
 chunks

30g soft brown sugar

2 tsp golden syrup

1 egg yolk, beaten

Butter, for greasing

Caster sugar, for dusting

1 small loaf sliced white bread, with
 the crusts cut off

28g butter, melted

Half-fat crème fraîche, to serve

Method

1 Put the water into a heavy-based pan, add the chunks of fruit and cook over a medium heat until soft.

2 Add the sugar and syrup. Remove from the heat and add the beaten egg.

3 Heat the oven to 220°C/425°F/Gas Mark 7. Lightly butter a Charlotte mould or 1.2 litre Pyrex dish and dust with a little caster sugar.

4 Cut the crustless bread into fingers and lightly dip them into the melted butter. Use the bread to line the sides of the mould or dish, making sure the bread overlaps slightly. Cut a circle the size of the bottom of the mould and line the base.

5 Fill the mould with the fruit and cover the top with another large circle of bread. Seal the joins with your fingers.

6 Cook the Charlotte for 10 minutes at the higher heat, then lower the temperature to 190°C/375°F/Gas Mark 5 for a further 40 minutes. Leave to cool first, then chill for about 4 hours. Serve with crème fraîche.

• • • • • • • • • •

Poached Cod in Caper Sauce with Lime Rice

Serves 4   Calories per Serving 304

Ingredients

4 skinless boneless cod fillets

1 teacup skimmed milk, for warming, and about two tablespoonsful, for mixing with flour

Seasoning, to taste

1 tbsp plain flour

28g butter

1 tsp grated lemon zest

2 tbsp capers

2 tbsp chopped parsley

2 tbsp half-fat crème fraîche

100g long-grain rice

Grated zest of 2 limes

Broccoli and French beans, to serve

Method

1 Place the cod fillets in a large frying-pan, add the milk and season with salt and pepper. Cover and poach gently for about 10 minutes until the fish is cooked through. Remove the fish and set aside, reserving the milk.

2 Add the flour to the warm milk, mixing a little with cold milk first to form a smooth paste. Stir constantly and add the butter and lemon zest.

3 Stir in the capers, parsley and crème fraîche. Season to taste with salt and pepper.

4 Meanwhile, cook the rice according to the instructions on the packet. Drain, and stir the lime zest into the rice.

5 Spoon the rice onto a warm serving dish. Top with the cod and pour the sauce over the top. Serve with broccoli and French beans.

Quorn & Pepper Kebabs

Serves 2   Calories per Serving 288

Ingredients

2 tbsp olive oil

Crushed sea salt

2 tsp dried chillies, crushed

450g Quorn, cubed

1 onion, cut into quarters

1 red, 1 green and 1 yellow pepper

900g broccoli, steamed and puréed

100g Basmati rice, steamed

Method

1 Heat a barbecue or grill until hot. In a bowl, combine the oil, sea salt and chillies. Add the Quorn and leave to marinate for 10 minutes.

2 Separate the layers of onion so that they form large pieces. Cut each pepper into 4 large pieces.

3 Start to load the ingredients onto skewers, alternating with Quorn, red pepper, onion, green pepper, Quorn, and so on, until all the ingredients are equally divided between the 4 skewers.

4 Spoon the remaining marinade over the kebabs, turning so that all the sides are coated. Make sure that the surfaces are covered with chillies.

5 Place on a rack over a grill pan and grill, turning frequently, until golden brown or chargrilled. Serve immediately on hot plates on a bed of hot broccoli purée with steamed rice.

Red Bean & Tomato Curry

Serves 4   Calories per Serving 102

Ingredients

2 tbsp sunflower oil

1 large onion, sliced

5 garlic cloves, crushed

1–2 fresh green chillies, cored, seeded and sliced

2.5cm (1in) piece of fresh root ginger, peeled and chopped

1 tsp curry powder

A pinch of cayenne pepper

Salt

½ tsp ground coriander

1 tsp turmeric

1 × 400g can chopped tomatoes

600g canned kidney beans

1 tbsp lemon juice

Fresh coriander leaves, to garnish

Method

1 Heat the sunflower oil in a large frying-pan, add the onion and garlic, chillies and ginger, and cook, stirring occasionally, until the onion is softened but not coloured.

2 Add the curry powder, cayenne pepper, salt to taste, ground coriander and turmeric and cook, stirring, for 2 minutes.

3 Add the tomatoes and most of their juice, and cook for about 3 minutes. Add the beans and cook for a further 5 minutes.

4 Add the lemon juice and serve hot, garnished with coriander leaves.

Roast Pineapple

Serves 4   Calories per Serving 108

Ingredients

1 whole pineapple

8 star anise

Half-fat crème fraîche or fromage frais, to serve

Method

1 Preheat the oven to 200°C/400°F/Gas Mark 6. Peel the pineapple and remove the central hard core. Alternatively, buy a whole fresh pineapple which is ready-prepared.

2 Stud the pineapple all over with the star anise. Cover tightly with foil and roast in the centre of the oven for 30 minutes.

3 Remove the pineapple from the oven and cut into large, 5-cm rings. Serve immediately with crème fraîche or fromage frais.

Salade Niçoise

Serves 2   Calories per Serving 326

Ingredients

2 tbsp olive oil

1 tbsp wine vinegar

2 leaves fresh mint, roughly crushed

Salad greens

8 small, waxy new potatoes, scrubbed, boiled and cooled

1 small tin tuna fish in brine, drained

100g French beans, steamed for 5 minutes and cooled

Small handful of black olives

2 hard-boiled eggs, shelled

Ground black pepper, to taste

Method

1 In a small jug, combine the oil and vinegar and add the mint leaves.

2 Arrange the salad greens on a serving plate, top with the potatoes, tuna and beans, then scatter the olives over the top. Quarter each hard-boiled egg and add to the salad.

3 Remove the mint from the dressing and pour over the salad just before serving. Season with black pepper.

Salmon Mousseline with Fresh Tomato Sauce

Serves 4   Calories per Serving 238

Ingredients

300g salmon fillet, skinned and cubed

1 clove garlic, chopped

1 egg

1 egg white

Seasoning, to taste

4 large tbsp half-fat crème fraîche

Butter, for greasing

Sauce

350g tomatoes, peeled and chopped

2 tbsp half-fat crème fraîche

2 tsp lemon juice

1 tbsp chopped dill

Sprig of dill, to garnish

French toast, to serve

Method

1 Preheat the oven to 180°C/350°F/Gas Mark 4. Place a roasting pan half full of very hot water into the oven.

2 Purée the salmon and garlic in a blender for 1 minute. Add the egg and egg white. Season, then mix again for a few seconds, then add the crème fraîche. Mix once again, but stop as soon as the mixture is thick and smooth. Leave to chill in the refrigerator.

3 Generously grease a 600-ml terrine or loaf tin. Spoon the mousseline inside and cover with a piece of greased foil. Place the terrine or tin inside the water bath and bake for 35 minutes or until the top is firm. Let cool.

4 Meanwhile, make the sauce by combining all the ingredients.

Turn the mousseline out onto a serving dish and slice. Pour the sauce around each slice.

5 Serve garnished with a sprig of dill, accompanied by freshly made thin French toast.

Smoked Salmon & Avocado Salad

Serves 2   Calories per Serving 273

Ingredients

Salad greens

Fresh vinaigrette dressing

2 slices smoked salmon

1 avocado pear

Juice and zest of one lime

Method

1 Place the salad greens onto a serving plate. Drizzle vinaigrette over the top. Slice the smoked salmon into thin strips and pile on top of the greens.

2 Peel the avocado pear and halve, removing the stone. Placing one half stone side down on a plate and slice horizontally. Gently press the avocado to one side so that it fans out. Repeat with the other avocado half.

3 Balance the avocado slices on top of the salmon and pour the lime juice over the top. Top with a sprinkling of lime zest.

Smoked Salmon on Potato Cakes

Serves 2   Calories per Serving 235

Ingredients

225g old potatoes, peeled

1 egg, beaten

100ml skimmed milk

Seasoning, to taste

2 tbsp white flour

8g butter, melted, and butter for
    greasing

Squeeze of lemon juice

2 slices smoked salmon

2 tbsp half-fat crème fraîche

A handful of chopped, fresh parsley

Method

1 Preheat the oven to 200°C/400°F/Gas Mark 6.

2 Boil and simmer the potatoes for about 20 minutes until done and then drain.

3 Add the egg and milk and mash well. Season and add the flour and use your hands to shape the mixture into 4 large potato balls.

4 Grease a baking sheet, and place the potato balls on it, flattening them to make large cakes. Brush with melted butter and bake in the centre of the oven for 25 minutes.

5 Meanwhile, cut the smoked salmon pieces into thin strips and toss in the lemon juice.

6 When the potato cakes are ready, remove from the oven and allow to cool slightly for 5 minutes. Divide the smoked salmon pieces between the four cakes and pile on top. Spoon 2–3 teaspoonsful of crème fraîche over the smoked salmon in mounds and top with a sprinkling of fresh parsley.

Spaghetti with Smoked Salmon & Dill

Serves 2   Calories per Serving 256

Ingredients

125g fresh spaghetti

2 tsp olive oil

1 clove garlic, crushed

50g smoked salmon, cut into strips

Seasoning, to taste

2 tbsp half-fat crème fraîche

1 fresh frond of dill, snipped, and one frond to garnish

Chopped fresh parsley, to garnish

Method

1 Cook the spaghetti in a pan of boiling water for 3 minutes or as directed on the package. Drain.

2 Heat the oil in a large frying-pan. Add the garlic and salmon, and cook for 30 seconds, stirring constantly.

3 Add the drained cooked spaghetti to the pan, heat through and season to taste.

4 Just before serving, add the crème fraîche and dill, and stir through quickly but do not apply heat. Turn straight onto hot plates, sprinkle with parsley and garnish with dill.

Note: This dish goes cold very quickly, so hot plates are essential.

Spiced Vegetable Risotto with Green Lentils

Serves 4   Calories per Serving 433

Ingredients

100g dried green lentils

1 large aubergine

2 courgettes

4 tbsp olive oil

1 tsp each: cumin, coriander seeds, paprika and garam masala

2 onions, sliced

4 cloves garlic, crushed

340g rice

150ml white wine or vermouth

900ml boiling water

2 tbsp green peppercorns

28g butter

50g fresh Parmesan, grated from block

Method

1 Simmer the lentils for about 20 minutes until soft. Drain and reserve. Preheat oven to 190°C/375°F/Gas Mark 5.

2 Cut the aubergine and courgettes into cubes.

3 Heat the oil in a heavy ovenproof pan and sauté the spices. Add the lentils and fry over medium heat until slightly brown. Then add the aubergine, courgettes, onions and garlic, and cook gently for about 4 minutes or until soft.

4 Add the rice, wine or vermouth, boiling water and peppercorns. Place in the oven and bake until the rice is cooked through, about 45 minutes.

5 Before serving, gently stir in the butter and grated Parmesan.

Spicy Cajun Chicken

Serves 4   Calories per Serving: 253 with rice, 154 with Salad

Ingredients

4 tsp citrus pepper

4 tsp coriander seeds

4 tsp cayenne pepper

4 tsp dried garlic granules

4 tsp dried onion granules

4 tsp dried chillies

4 skinless, boneless, chicken breasts, slightly flattened

3–4 tbsp olive oil

200g cooked rice or a selection of dressed salad leaves, to serve

Method

1 Combine all the spices and flavourings.

2 Lightly brush the chicken with oil. Press spice and flavourings mixture into the chicken breasts to cover all surfaces.

3 Heat the remaining oil in a large frying-pan. Add the chicken and sauté gently until cooked thoroughly, turning every few minutes. Turn up the heat and sear the chicken.

4 Serve immediately on hot rice, cutting the chicken breasts diagonally into thick slices. Alternatively, serve on a bed of dressed salad leaves.

Spicy Yoghurt-baked Chicken

Serves 2   Calories per Serving 275

Ingredients

1 carton live, plain bio yoghurt

Juice of 1 fresh lime

A little fresh ginger root, grated

A few fennel seeds

1 tsp each: cumin, turmeric and cayenne pepper

1 clove garlic, crushed

2 skinless, boneless chicken breasts

125g Basmati rice

Green salad, to serve

Method

1 To prepare the marinade, combine the yoghurt, lime juice, ginger, fennel seeds, spices and garlic in a bowl and mix thoroughly.

2 Place the chicken in the marinade, coat completely, cover and set aside for 2–8 hours.

3 Preheat the oven to 180°C/350°F/Gas Mark 4. Remove the chicken from the marinade and place in an ovenproof dish, cover and bake in the oven for 25 minutes. Spread the marinade sauce over the chicken and return to the oven for a further 20 minutes.

4 Boil the rice as directed on the packet and drain. Serve the chicken on a bed of rice with a green salad.

Spinach & Avocado Salad

Serves 4   Calories per Serving 290

Ingredients

450g young leaf spinach

2 ripe avocados

2 tbsp hazelnut oil

2 tsp wine vinegar

Seasoning, to taste

85g hazelnuts, coarsely chopped

Crusty French bread, to serve

Method

1 Remove the stalks from the spinach leaves, wash and pat dry.

2 Peel, stone and slice the avocados.

3 Mix the oil, vinegar and seasoning in a bowl. Add the avocados and spinach and sprinkle with hazelnuts.

4 Toss the salad lightly at the table, making sure that the avocado does not break up. Serve with crusty French bread.

Stir-fry Chicken with Carrot & Orange Salad

Serves 4   Calories per Serving 220

Ingredients

2 skinless, boneless chicken breasts

2 tsp dried chillies

2 tbsp vegetable oil

Fresh watercress

2 oranges

2 carrots

Soy sauce, to taste

Method

1 Cut the chicken breasts into thin strips. Sprinkle the dried chillies onto a small plate and roll the chicken in them until

lightly coated. Press the chicken into the chillies, if necessary, to make them stick.

2 Heat the oil in a large frying-pan and gently fry the chicken, turning quickly at first to seal. Cover the pan and lower the heat to cook the chicken.

3 Sprinkle watercress over a serving dish to cover the surface. Remove the zest from the oranges and reserve. Peel the oranges and cut into segments.

4 With a potato peeler, peel the carrots lengthwise to form long strips. (These should curl slightly to form 'ribbons'.) Combine with the orange segments and pile onto the watercress bed.

5 Check that the chicken is cooked by cutting into a strip of meat. The flesh should be white throughout without a hint of pink. Turn up the heat to brown.

6 Add the grated orange zest and a good dash of soy sauce. Combine well, then turn straight onto the top of the salad and serve immediately.

Strawberry & Cucumber Salad

Serves 4   Calories per Serving 73

Ingredients

Lamb's lettuce or watercress

450g strawberries, hulled

1 whole cucumber, peeled

2 tbsp hazelnut oil

1 tbsp raspberry vinegar

A few mint leaves, crushed

Cold chicken or ham, to serve

Method

1 Line a decorative serving dish with lamb's lettuce or watercress.

2 Slice the strawberries very thinly and place them in a bowl.

3 Using the long-slice part of a grater, hold the cucumber so

• • • • • • • • • •

that it is facing downwards and grate long strips down its length to form 'ribbons'. Avoid the seeds in the middle of the cucumber and work round until only the seeds are left. Discard.

4 Combine the cucumber 'ribbons' with the strawberries and pile onto the watercress or lamb's lettuce.

5 Mix all the dressing ingredients together separately, including the mint leaves, shake well and leave to stand until just before serving. Discard the mint before pouring. Do not toss the salad. Serve with cold chicken or ham.

Sweet & Sour Vegetables with Rice

Serves 4   Calories per Serving 223

Ingredients

4 tbsp vegetable oil	1 tbsp malt vinegar
1 onion, chopped finely	1 tbsp soy sauce
4 courgettes, sliced	1 tbsp each sultanas and almonds
100g French beans	1 tsp crushed cloves
8 baby sweetcorn	2 tbsp honey
200g mushrooms, sliced	Seasoning, to taste
2 carrots, chopped into batons	Boiled rice, to serve

Method

1 Heat the oil in a large frying-pan and cook the onion until soft. Add the rest of the vegetables and stir well. Cook for 5 minutes.

2 Add all the other ingredients, stir well and cook through for a further 3 minutes. Serve with boiled rice.

Szechuan Pepper & Tofu Stir-fry

Serves 4   Calories per Serving 288

Ingredients

3 tbsp vegetable oil

1 × 285g pack tofu, drained and cut into cubes

1 tsp Chinese 5-spice powder

¼ tsp chilli powder

1 red pepper, de-seeded and cut into strips

1 bunch salad onions, trimmed and sliced diagonally

2 tsp cornflour

1 tbsp dark soy sauce

1 tbsp dry sherry

2 tbsp dark brown sugar

4 tbsp water

1 tsp sesame seeds, toasted

2 sheets egg noodles

Method

1 Heat 1 tbsp of the oil in a large frying-pan, add the tofu and fry for 1–2 minutes, until brown. Remove and drain.

2 In a bowl, mix the spices with the tofu. Heat the remaining oil, add the pepper and spring onions, and stir-fry.

3 Combine the cornflour, soy sauce, sherry, sugar and water, and add to the vegetables. Cook for a further 2 minutes, stirring until thickened.

4 Add the sesame seeds and the tofu to the vegetable mixture and heat gently for a further 1–2 minutes.

5 Cook the noodles according to the instructions on the package, drain and combine with the tofu mixture. Serve immediately on hot plates.

Tofu Sticks with Spicy Spinach

Serves 2   Calories per Serving 230

Ingredients

1 tbsp vegetable oil

200g packet frozen spinach, thawed

1 green chilli, finely chopped

1 tsp chilli powder, plus a little for
  dusting

200g tofu, rinsed and cut into cubes

1 red and green pepper, cut into
  quarters

8 slices onion, cut suitably for
  threading onto skewers

2 tsp sesame seeds, toasted

Salt and coarsely-ground black pepper

Method

1 Preheat grill or barbecue to hot.

2 Put 1 tbsp oil into a large frying-pan over a gentle heat and fry the spinach with the chopped chillies and the chilli powder for 1–2 minutes. Remove, drain and keep warm in an oven-proof dish.

3 Thread the tofu cubes, the pepper quarters and the onion onto two skewers, alternating them. Brush or drizzle over the other tablespoon of oil, making sure all sides are coated.

4 Grill for 5 minutes, turning frequently and making sure the kebabs do not burn. Brush with any remaining or a little extra oil to prevent them drying out. Finally, dust with a little chilli powder before continuing to grill for a further minute.

5 Turn the kebabs onto the hot spinach mixture and sprinkle with the toasted sesame seeds to serve.

Two-Pear Salad

Serves 4   Calories per Serving 105

This dish works best with chargrilled salmon or white fish, or large chargrilled prawns.

Ingredients

1 large, ripe dessert pear	1 tbsp raspberry vinegar
1 large, ripe avocado pear	1 tsp sugar
Juice of 1 lemon	Coarsely ground black pepper
2 tbsp olive oil	

Method

1 Peel the pear, slice into quarters and remove the core. Slice carefully into thin slices.

2 Cut the avocado pear in two, remove the stone and peel each half. Cut into thin slices.

3 Interleave the slices on a round serving dish, alternating pear with avocado to form a wheel. Squeeze lemon juice over the top to prevent browning.

4 Mix the dressing ingredients together and, just before serving, drizzle over the top.

Waldorf Salad

Serves 2   Calories per Serving 200

Ingredients

1 red apple, sliced	12 walnuts, crushed into pieces
2 celery sticks, cut into 2-cm strips	1 tbsp good mayonnaise
20 grapes, halved	Lettuce leaves

• • • • • • • • •

Method

1 Place the apple and celery in a bowl.

2 Add the grapes and walnuts. Bind with the mayonnaise and mix well.

3 Turn out onto the bed of lettuce on a serving plate and serve.

Warm Chicken Salad

Serves 2   Calories per Serving 238

This is an incredibly quick and easy dish to make. It is low-calorie and full of goodness for any dieter. Have different spices at the ready to vary the taste.

Ingredients

Selection of dried spices or herbs, to taste

1 skinless, boneless chicken breast, cut into thin strips *or*

200g bought chicken strips, cut for stir-frying

Packet of bought Bistro-style or Nantaise salad (lamb's lettuce and grated beetroot)

½ carrot, grated

½ courgette, grated

1 tbsp sweetcorn

1 tbsp pine kernels (optional)

1 tbsp soy sauce (optional)

1 tbsp good-quality French dressing (not low-fat)

Method

1 Place 2 teaspoons of your chosen spice or herb mixture on a small plate. Roll the chicken pieces in them until they are coated evenly.

2 Arrange the salad on a serving plate. Make a bed of Salade Nantaise leaves and top with the carrot, courgette and sweetcorn.

3 Toast the pine kernels by placing them in a frying-pan with 1 teaspoon of oil and cook over a medium heat for several

• • • • • • • • •

minutes. Cover the pan and keep shaking. Check when the pine kernels have turned brown and toasted, remove from the heat and turn out onto a kitchen towel. Reserve.

4 Heat the rest of the oil in a frying-pan and add the chicken pieces. Keep the heat low and turn several times until the chicken has turned white on the outside. Cover the pan and leave to cook for a further 5 minutes.

5 Turn up the heat to brown the chicken, add the soy sauce, if using, and flash fry for a further 1–2 minutes. Turn immediately onto the salad, dress with vinaigrette and toss the toasted pine kernels over the top to serve.

Winter Salad

Serves 4   Calories per Serving 170

Ingredients

2 red apples, grated including skin

1 courgette, grated including peel

Juice of one lemon

Quarter of a white cabbage, finely chopped or grated

2 large carrots, peeled and grated

Quarter of a red cabbage, finely chopped or grated

50g dried sultanas

50g walnut pieces (optional)

4 tbsp vinaigrette

Jacket potatoes and cheese, to serve

Method

1 Put the apples and courgette into a bowl and squeeze lemon juice over them to prevent browning.

2 Add all the other vegetables, dried sultanas and walnuts, and mix well. Just before serving, add the vinaigrette and toss. Transfer to a salad bowl. Serve with jacket potatoes and cheese.

• • • • • • • • • •

Monica's Mailbag

Let me know how you are getting on, tell me what problems you have and share with me how successful you have been getting back into your jeans! Write to me at:

Monica's Mailbag
PO Box 58
Oxon OX12 9BS

If you'd like a reply, please enclose a stamped self-addressed envelope.

• • • • • • • • • •

If you think the **Get Back Into Your Jeans Diet**
was good, just WAIT until you read
Monica Grenfall's two other great diet books!

Fabulous in a Fortnight

Every woman, from sixteen to ninety, has what it takes to look good – because that something comes from within. All you need to learn is how to make the most of yourself. And it needn't take a month or a miracle – just follow Monica Grenfell's fantastic two-week plan!

Looking forward to a wedding, special family occasion or beach holiday? Getting ready for an important job interview? Monica's day-by-day countdown includes an easy-to-follow diet plan, simple exercise routines for toning and beauty tips – plus checklists for all the embarrasing little things you mightn't have thought of. Start today, and in just a fortnight you'll be looking sensational for any event where you need to look your best.

'Best class I've ever been to'
The Sun

Get your copy of **Fabulous in a Fortnight**,
Monica's all-body diet and beauty plan, today!

• • • • • • • • • •

5 Days to a Flatter Stomach

Are you always on a diet? Do you reach your goal weight only to find your stomach is still big? Are you fed up with diets which leave you bloated and uncomfortable?

This breakthrough books shows you how in just FIVE DAYS you can lose weight and inches round your stomach, by banishing bloat, improving muscle tone and reducing fat.

This affordable regime gives you a five-day plan, with an easy-to-follow maintenance diet for the future and recipes the whole family can enjoy. Read the real-life stories of women who followed the plan and were thrilled with the results.

5 Days to a Flatter Stomach is available
through all good bookshops, or by using the
order form overleaf.

• • • • • • • • • •

Pan and Boxtree books are available from your local bookshop. Ask for details of Monica Grenfell's latest book!

Fabulous in a Fortnight

Demy pb 0330 35368 3 £7.99

5 Days to a Flatter Stomach

B pb 07522 2130 2 £4.99

Alternatively send a cheque or postal order payable to:

Book Services By Post
PO Box 29
Douglas, Isle of Man
IM99 1BQ

Or call 01624 675137 with a major credit card number. Postage and packing free!

• • • • • • • • • •